SURGICAL FINALS
Passing the Clinical

Third Edition

John SP Lumley MS FRCS

Emeritus Professor of Vascular Surgery,
University of London,
Hon C S Great Ormond Street Hospital, London
Past Council Member and Chairman of Examiners,
Primary Fellowship Examiners, Royal College of Surgeons, England

Petrut Gogalniceanu MBBS BSc MRCS

Specialist Registrar in General Surgery,
London Deanery,
London

Gina R Kuperberg BSc MBBS(Hons), PhD

Professor of Cognitive Neuroscience,
Massachusetts General Hospital and Tufts University,
Boston, MA.

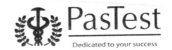

PasTest
Dedicated to your success

© 2011 PasTest Ltd
Knutsford Cheshire WA16 8DX
Telephone: 01565 752000

First published 1996
Second edition 2003
Reprinted 2005, 2009
Third edition 2011

ISBN 1 905635 71 0
ISBN 978 1 905635 71 9

A catalogue record for this book is available from the British Library.

The information contained within this book was obtained by the authors from reliable sources. However, while every effort has been made to ensure its accuracy, no responsibility for loss, damage or injury occasioned to any person acting or refraining from action as a result of information contained herein can be accepted by the publishers or authors.

PasTest Revision Books, Intensive Courses and Online Revision

PasTest has been established in the field of undergraduate and postgraduate medical education since 1972, providing revision books, intensive study courses and online revision for doctors preparing for their professional examinations.

Books and courses are available for:

Medical undergraduates, MRCGP, MRCP Parts 1 and 2, MRCPCH Parts 1 and 2, MRCS, MRCOG Parts 1 and 2, DRCOG, DCH, FRCA, Dentistry.

For further details contact:

PasTest, Freepost, Knutsford, Cheshire WA16 7BR

Tel: 01565 752000   **Fax: 01565 650264**

www.pastest.co.uk   **enquiries@pastest.co.uk**

Typeset by Carnegie Book Production, Lancaster
Printed and bound in the UK by CPI Anthony Rowe

CONTENTS

PREFACE

History and examination are essential parts of clinical practice and key elements in medical training, requiring constant supervision and evaluation. The assessment of these skills is therefore a mandatory requirement of every medical school. The form of this assessment varies: continuous assessment is common, and desirable, with constructive feedback, to ensure that students are developing appropriate skills.

As students approach their summative assessments and final examinations, however, examiners have a responsibility to ensure that candidates are competent to progress independently and that patient safety is assured. Although symptoms and signs and their clinical interpretation do not change markedly, their forms of assessment have evolved into structured, consistent, reliable and measurable methods, ensuring that specific skills are examined and achieved by every successful candidate.

The primary aim of this text is to reduce the chances of failure in the clinical part of surgical finals. This is by encompassing the core knowledge and skills needed to pass finals, and providing a reliable and safe approach to patients and their surgical problems; it also addresses the requirements of the various forms of assessment that are in current use. Student as well as staff involvement in the initiation and development of the first and subsequent editions has retained a close link to teaching and assessment methods, and most importantly to clinical practice.

The text takes the candidate through the clinical history and examination of frequently encountered surgical conditions and common written or verbal questions that are added to manned or unmanned examination stations. The emphasis is surgical and topics more pertinent to medical specialities, such as cardiac, respiratory, neurology, dermatology and psychiatry, are not included. For these and other aspects of finals, consult the companion Medical, OSCE and EMQ volumes.

We hope that the continued popularity of the text reflects its close link to the examination systems across the UK and reader's success in his or her surgical finals.

INTRODUCTION

By the end of your undergraduate training you will have probably accumulated enough knowledge and clinical experience to pass finals; however, clear organisation of factual material and refining of your clinical skills increases your confidence, reduces examination stress and ensures optimal performance. This book addresses the clinical aspects of the examination in a concise, ordered and meaningful way, presenting essential information in a form that is linked to the various examination systems that are in current use across the UK.

The book covers the following:

- How to prepare for your surgical clinical examination

- How to take a history and examine a patient with a surgical problem

- Schematic approaches to all common surgical conditions

- The likely surgical stations that you will encounter in OSCEs

- The long and short cases that you are likely to encounter, with lists of features, tables of differential diagnoses and treatment

- Frequently asked questions in all forms of surgical examination

- An answer section to frequently asked questions

- The approach to vivas

- A checklist against which to plan your revision

The emphasis of the book is on a practical approach to clinical problems. The techniques described are applicable to the final examination and will keep your examiner happy. Make sure that you know the format of the examination in your own school, the emphasis on long or short cases, and the form and usual content of OSCEs – match your use of the text to this style. The concise, dogmatic and 'no-frills' approach has been taken to allow rapid retrieval and packaging of information to your needs: the aim at all times is to minimise your examination difficulties.

SYLLABUS CHECKLIST

As an aid to revision, use this syllabus as your own personal checklist. Page numbers are given in brackets after each case. You should aim to achieve at least two ticks per case before the date of the examination. If you have not actually seen a condition, look it up in an illustrated textbook.

	Read	Seen Taught on	Happy with
General examination and pain (25)	☐	☐	☐
Swellings and ulcers			
1. Squamous cell papilloma / skin tag (46)	☐	☐	☐
2. Wart (46)	☐	☐	☐
3. Seborrhoeic keratosis / senile wart (46)	☐	☐	☐
4. Pigmented naevus or malignant melanoma (47)	☐	☐	☐
5. Dermatofibroma / histiocytoma (47)	☐	☐	☐
6. Pyogenic granuloma (48)	☐	☐	☐
7. Keloid or hypertrophic scar (48)	☐	☐	☐
8. Keratoacanthoma / molluscum sebaceum (49)	☐	☐	☐
9. Keratin horn (49)	☐	☐	☐
10. Sebaceous cyst (49)	☐	☐	☐
11. Boil or carbuncle (50)	☐	☐	☐
12. Hydradenitis suppurativa (50)	☐	☐	☐
13. Strawberry naevus (51)	☐	☐	☐
14. Port-wine stain (51)	☐	☐	☐
15. Lipoma (52)	☐	☐	☐
16. Dermoid cyst (52)	☐	☐	☐

		Read	Seen Taught on	Happy with
17.	Ganglion (52)	☐	☐	☐
18.	Ulcer with a sloping edge (54)	☐	☐	☐
19.	Ulcer with a punched-out edge (54)	☐	☐	☐
20.	Ulcer with a raised edge (55)	☐	☐	☐
	Neck swellings and thyroid lumps	☐	☐	☐
1.	Goitre (68)	☐	☐	☐
2.	Thyroglossal cyst (71)	☐	☐	☐
3.	Cervical lymphadenopathy (73)	☐	☐	☐
4.	Salivary gland swelling (74)	☐	☐	☐
5.	Cervical rib (76)	☐	☐	☐
6.	Carotid body tumour (77)	☐	☐	☐
7.	Branchial cyst / sinus / fistula (78)	☐	☐	☐
	The breast			
1.	Breast carcinoma (88)	☐	☐	☐
2.	Fibroadenoma (91)	☐	☐	☐
3.	Fibroadenosis (91)	☐	☐	☐
4.	Nipple discharge (92)	☐	☐	☐
	The gastrointestinal tract			
	Scars and stomas (105)	☐	☐	☐
1.	Hepatomegaly (107)	☐	☐	☐
2.	Splenomegaly (108)	☐	☐	☐
3.	Hepatosplenomegaly (109)	☐	☐	☐
4.	Enlarged kidneys (109)	☐	☐	☐

		Read	Seen Taught on	Happy with
5.	Mass in the right hypochondrium (111)	☐	☐	☐
6.	Mass in the epigastrium (112)	☐	☐	☐
7.	Mass in the left hypochondrium (113)	☐	☐	☐
8.	Mass in the right loin (113)	☐	☐	☐
9.	Mass in the umbilical region (113)	☐	☐	☐
10.	Mass in the left loin (113)	☐	☐	☐
11.	Mass in the right iliac fossa (114)	☐	☐	☐
12.	Mass in the left iliac fossa (115)	☐	☐	☐
13.	Abdominal distension (116)	☐	☐	☐

Lump in the groin

1.	Inguinal hernia (129)	☐	☐	☐
2.	Femoral hernia (132)	☐	☐	☐
3.	Saphena varix (133)	☐	☐	☐
4.	Femoral aneurysm (133)	☐	☐	☐
5.	Lymph nodes (133)	☐	☐	☐
6.	Psoas abscess (134)	☐	☐	☐

Urology

1.	Suprapubic mass (140)	☐	☐	☐

Scrotal and inguinal

1.	Testicular tumour (142)	☐	☐	☐
2.	Varicocele (143)	☐	☐	☐
3.	Hydrocele (143)	☐	☐	☐
4.	Epididymal cyst (145)	☐	☐	☐
5.	Absent testis in a child (145)	☐	☐	☐

		Read	Seen Taught on	Happy with
8.	Mallet finger (197)	☐	☐	☐
9.	Boutonnière deformity (197)	☐	☐	☐
10.	Swan-neck deformity (197)	☐	☐	☐
11.	Trigger finger / stenosing tenosynovitis (198)	☐	☐	☐
12.	Rheumatoid arthritis (198)	☐	☐	☐
13.	Osteoarthritis (199)	☐	☐	☐
14.	The wasted hand (199)	☐	☐	☐
15.	Fall on an outstretched hand (FOOSH) (200)	☐	☐	☐
16.	Shoulder injuries (201)	☐	☐	☐
17.	Hallux valgus (bunions) (202)	☐	☐	☐
18.	Hammer toe (202)	☐	☐	☐
19.	Claw toes (202)	☐	☐	☐
	Arterial insufficiency of the lower limb	☐	☐	☐
1.	Intermittent claudication (213)	☐	☐	☐
2.	Rest pain / critical ischaemia (217)	☐	☐	☐
3.	Diabetic foot (217)	☐	☐	☐
4.	Aortic aneurysm (218)	☐	☐	☐
5.	Amputation (219)	☐	☐	☐
	Venous disorders of the lower limb	☐	☐	☐
1.	Varicose veins (227)	☐	☐	☐
2.	Venous insufficiency (229)	☐	☐	☐
3.	AV malformations (229)	☐	☐	☐

	Read	Seen Taught on	Happy with
Neurology (232)	☐	☐	☐
The postoperative patient (239)	☐	☐	☐

ACKNOWLEDGEMENTS

To Marcia and Louis Kuperberg

To Calina, Dan, Mocoo,
Teodora and Flory"

Thanks to Sophie Lumley

We would also like to thank Mr James Pegrum (MRCS, BSc MSc) for his specialist review of the orthopaedic section of this new edition which included the following chapters (Joint, hands, hip, knee, foot and ankle)

ABBREVIATIONS

The following abbreviations have been used throughout this book

ABG	arterial blood gases
ACTH	adrenocorticotropic hormone
ALP	alkaline phosphatase
ALT	alanine aminotransferase
ANA	antinuclear factor
ASIS	anterior superior iliac spine
ATLS	Advanced Trauma Life Support
AV	arteriovenous
CLL	chronic lymphocytic leukaemia
CRP	C-reactive protein
CSF	cerebrospinal fluid
CT	computed tomography
DIP(J)	distal interphalangeal (joint)
DVT	deep vein thrombosis
ECG	electrocardiogram
ENT	ear, nose and throat
ESR	erythrocyte sedimentation rate
FBC	full blood count
GCS	Glasgow coma scale
GI(T)	gastrointestinal (tract)
HIV	human immunodeficiency virus
HRT	hormone replacement therapy
IP(J)	interphalangeal (joint)
JVP	jugular venous pressure

LFT	liver function test
MCP(J)	metacarpophalangeal (joint)
MRI	magnetic resonance imaging
NSAID	non-steroidal anti-inflammatory drug
PIP(J)	proximal interphalangeal (joint)
RIF	right iliac fossa
T_3	triiodothyronine
T_4	thyroxine
TB	tuberculosis
TFT	thyroid function test
TNM	tumour / node / metastases (classification)
TSH	thyroid-stimulating hormone
WBC	white blood cell (count)

Section 1
General points

The clinical: examiners, patients and preparation

FORMAT

The examiners

Examiners of a long case traditionally work in pairs. There is normally one 'internal' examiner (from your own teaching hospital) and one 'external' (invited from outside). The difficulty in finding enough clinical material to assess large numbers of candidates has led to the merging of medical and surgical cases and an increase in assessments of structures. However, the text has been structured to be applicable to all forms of assessment.

You will usually be told who your examiners are. It is worth knowing their special interests, even though their questions will not be confined to these areas. Talk to medical students who have been taught by your examiners to find out any particular preferences in examination technique (eg always kneeling down to examine the abdomen).

The patients

The range of conditions that you will see in the examination is not necessarily representative of the conditions seen in general hospital care. First, you will never be given a very ill patient with, for example, an acute abdomen or an acutely ischaemic limb. Second, there are some rare conditions that crop up disproportionately in examinations: such patients usually have long-standing problems with good physical signs. Examples are AV malformations or carotid body tumours.

Patients are drawn from four sources: inpatients, patients coming up from clinics, 'professional' patients and simulated patients.

1. Inpatients

Most inpatients transferred to the examination will be awaiting operations such as hernia repairs or removal of breast lumps. Postoperative patients are also available for the clinicals: after all, you will be expected to manage such patients in your F1 and F2 years. A minority of patients will be those recovering from acute conditions, with good histories and/or physical signs that have not yet resolved.

2. Patients coming up from clinics

Patients with good physical signs who attend clinics in the few weeks before the clinicals are often asked to come up for the examination. Try to attend clinics in your hospital in the lead-up to finals. (For example, before surgical finals, one of the authors walked into the examination centre with a fellow candidate who pointed out two patients who she recognised: 'He has a sebaceous cyst on his forehead. She's got a left submandibular tumour.' After revising these two conditions, she was given both patients as short cases!)

3. 'Professional' patients

These are patients with long-standing signs who are listed on a computer database and who have been called up numerous times in the past. Such patients are usually excellent historians and may even point out their physical signs.

4. Simulated patients

Simulated patients are healthy individuals who are trained to simulate a patient's illness in a standard manner. They are usually actors. Some training is usually required to ensure that they are able to bring out the main points in the history on request and within the time allowed. Simulated patients can become skilled historians and very persuasive patients, such as when replicating a psychiatric disturbance. They are often asked to give their own marks on the student encounter.

In addition a video of a patient presenting a history can be shown.

PREPARATION

Early preparation

Don't fall into bad habits

Ask a doctor to watch you examine and listen to your presentations as early and as often as possible. Without this, it is very easy to acquire bad habits that are difficult to break.

Act as a chaperone

Senior medical students in their clinical years are often used as 'chaperones' in clinical examinations. Their role is to escort the candidates from room to room, ring the bells and ensure that the examination runs smoothly. If you are given this opportunity, take it. You will get an idea of the examination format and there will often be time to examine the patients yourselves afterwards. There can be no better preparation: some of the same patients may even come up the following year.

The revision period

Team up with a colleague

As the examination draws closer, pair up with a fellow student whose aims and standards are similar to your own and whose opinion you respect. By working in pairs, each of you can act as an examiner in turn, covering long and short cases and talking through topics that could arise in vivas. Remember that each person works at his or her own pace and thinks that the other knows more than him- or herself. The relationship should be mutually beneficial.

Ask for senior help

During the revision period don't hesitate to ask for extra teaching from senior staff: they've all been through finals themselves and are usually glad to help. Don't be put off by any tendency to teach by humiliation and don't worry if you are given different information or conflicting approaches: just extract what you consider the best information from each teacher.

Bleep the FY1 and FY2 and ask for lists of patients to see as long and short cases. Ask when patients are to be admitted. Also find out when day surgery lists take place: here you will find many swellings, ulcers, varicose veins and hernias to examine.

Revise efficiently

This book gives plenty of lists of clinical features and provides tables of differential diagnoses. Modify these to make your own lists: you will remember best what you compile yourself. Laptops or card systems may be a useful revision aid at this stage.

Try not to work late into the night, relax before you go to bed, avoid excess coffee and keep up physical exercise. You will retain much more if you are alert during the revision period than if you are exhausted. Remember that hypnotics and anxiolytics can dull your mind on the day of the examination: take them only under medical supervision.

2

The OSLER/ long case

Long cases in finals may be combined medical and surgical assessment with one or two examiners. You may or may not be observed during the history and examination. Often you are taken back to a patient to demonstrate specific signs.

The traditional long case format has inherent problems of objectivity and reliability. In response to such problems, standardised patients and markings systems have been introduced. These include the introduction of the 'objective structured long examination record' (OSLER). The OSLER might include more than one case (a real patient, a simulated patient or a video, see page 4), each allocated 20–30 minutes, usually with a single examiner. This allows the examiner to test specific aspects of knowledge, skills or management decisions. Shorter periods may be allotted to specific parts of the history taking or focal examination.

Allocating your time

Be sure that you know well in advance how much time you will be given for the long case. This varies from school to school. Normally, 20 minutes is the minimum. This provides very little time for complex peripheral vascular or GIT problems; listen to or read the instructions very carefully. If it looks as if the history will take longer than half the allotted time, start examining after you have taken the details of the presenting complaint and past medical history. The remainder of the history can be taken at convenient points during the examination. It is essential that you practise this.

Rapport with the patient

It is important to establish a good rapport with your patient. Be friendly and polite. Introduce yourself and say what you wish to do (I am ...., I am a medical student and I would like to ask you about and examine your ....); ask for their verbal consent to these procedures (Are you happy with this?). Make sure that the patient is comfortable at all times. Do not ask the diagnosis immediately. On the other hand, if you gain the patient's sympathy, he or she may point you in the right direction and may even show you physical signs.

The history

Go through your usual scheme, which should be familiar by now. You will probably be given paper and a writing board. Start with name, age, occupation and marital status. This is followed by seven headings.

1. Presenting complaint

Ask about the main problem(s). List these together with a time scale, eg

- Abdominal pain: 3 weeks

- Nausea: 4 days

2. History of presenting complaint

Always include the systemic enquiry of the system relevant to the presenting complaint. Also ask the other appropriate questions (revised in sections of this book).

3. Past medical and surgical history

When asking about previous surgery, remember to ask if there were any problems with the anaesthetic, and how long the patient was in hospital.

4. Drug history and allergies (including recreational drugs)

5. Family history

Again, include questions about anaesthetic reactions.

6. Social history

A good social history will make you stand out from other candidates. Don't just ask about alcohol and smoking; check environmental hazards (eg asbestos exposure). It is important that you know how well the patient will manage at home during the postoperative period. Therefore ask about family, neighbours, carers, GP home visits, district nurses, home help, meals on wheels and financial problems.

Your social history should be relevant to the patient's problem, so if you have a patient with a stoma, enquire into the details of stoma care, and whether they can change the bag themself. If you have a patient with an orthopaedic problem or amputation, ask about physiotherapy, occupational therapy, aids and appliances.

7. Systemic enquiry

As in subsequent sections.

The examination

Your hands should be washed clean and warm before commencing any examination. (For more than one station there will usually be an alcohol wash at the bedside; if not, ask an attendant where you can wash your hands.) Your examination may be observed by an examiner. This does not mean that you should change your clinical approach: the order for general and regional examination is just the same, as outlined in the text, and the one you have practised with supervisors and your chosen colleague (page 5).

Start your examination by forming a general impression of the patient: observing him or her from the **end of the bed**. If you are being monitored by an examiner, state what you are doing and comment on the presence or absence of the signs that you are looking for. Next move to the **patient's right-hand side** (this is not only a time-honoured tradition, but also efficient [even if you are left handed] – manoeuvres in this text are described from this position).

Look for JACCOL (**j**aundice, **a**naemia, **c**yanosis, **c**lubbing, **o**edema, **l**ymphadenopathy) and examine the hands. In your systems approach pay particular attention to the system relevant to the presenting complaint. However, aim to be thorough; always take the pulse and blood pressure. Remember to test the urine. A dipstick should be provided.

Observation, palpation, percussion and auscultation will have been repeatedly drummed into you by your teachers, and look, feel, move and measure for joints – this is not the time to forget them! When palpating, always watch your patient's face for distress, and apologise for causing any discomfort. When auscultating, warm the bell or diaphragm and tap the end to make sure that you are plugged into the right bit before you start.

An examiner may ask what you are doing at each stage; take this into account when you are preparing with a colleague and do likewise. When you have finished your examination make sure that the patient is covered and comfortable.

Thinking time

If you are not being observed you will usually have a few minutes between examining the patient and presenting your findings. During this time, reorganise any misplaced information and summarise the case in writing. You might also predict your examiners' questions so that you are one step ahead. The sections on 'typical cases' in this book will help you to do this.

Presenting your findings

The examiners will usually tell you what they want. Normally they will ask you to tell them about the patient who you have just seen. They may add a rider such as 'stick to the important features'. Don't get flustered if they start with 'What's the diagnosis?'

If your patient was a poor historian, start by commenting on this fact: this is an important sign in itself and allowances will be made. However, it is no excuse for a poor presentation.

Your presentation should be as concise, snappy and comprehensive as possible. Place your notes in front of you for reference but talk, don't read, to the examiners. Don't panic if your notes are taken away from you: the history and examination will be fresh in your mind and you will remember more than you think.

If the patient has more than one complaint this should be brought out by listing the presenting complaints. Then explain, 'I will describe each of these in turn.'

You should not give long lists of negative findings: if the main problem is abdominal and you have found no other abnormality, it is quite permissible to state that 'other systems are normal'.

The examiners may interrupt you in the middle of your presentation. They may be happy with the way that you have started and want to go on to the next point, they may wish to discuss a problem in more depth, or they may simply be bored after listening to several well-delivered histories in a row.

You may be taken back to the patient to demonstrate an abnormal finding. This does not necessarily mean that there is any doubt about your findings: you may have elicited a sign previously missed! At the end of your presentation give the diagnosis (if you are sure of it), and/or list the common differentials or causes of the patient's problem.

3 The OSCEs and short cases

Objective structured clinical examination (OSCE) assesses a broad range of knowledge and skills in a quantifiable, valid and reliable form. The OSCE aims to assess your factual recall, your interpretative skills, your decision making, your behavioural attitude in professional practice and your ability to perform particular practical tasks. It ensures that each of you is presented with the same material and therefore provides a uniform evaluation and marking system.

The OSCE often includes short cases. These are probably the most difficult part of the clinical examination because you will be required to examine a patient under the eagle eye of one or two examiners. The examiners will watch for three things.

1. A caring and competent approach

You should always introduce yourself, say what you would like to do and ask permission (see page 8). Fully expose the part of the body that you wish to examine. Remember to compare both sides: if the examiner tells you to examine one leg, always expose the other leg as well. However, keep the patient 'decent', eg when exposing the legs, cover the groin. Before palpation, never forget to ask if there is any tenderness. The patient should be comfortable at all times. Thank the patient and cover him or her up before presenting your findings.

2. A good examination technique

Your examination of the short cases should be a smooth, thorough and slick performance. The only way to achieve this is to practise again and again so that the routine becomes second nature. Find a colleague to work with and examine under observed and, whenever possible, supervised conditions.

Note the following points:

- Do not take the examination schemes provided in this book as gospel. Modify them according to your own teaching and individual preference.

- Don't be such an automaton that you fail to listen to the instruction: if the examiner tells you to 'palpate the abdomen', do not start with the hands.

- Passing the short cases is rather like passing a driving test: you must actually *show* your examiners that you are following the correct routine, eg by standing at the end of the bed to observe the patient.

- Although you are not supposed to take a history during the short case, you *are* allowed certain questions, eg before examining a lump you cannot see, ask the patient to point out its exact position.

Three further questions that should be asked regarding a lump are: Is it tender/painful (before you start)? How long have you had it? Is it changing in size?

There are certain things that you are not expected to include in the examination situation, such as a rectal examination. However, you *must* indicate to the examiners that you would normally examine these areas. Furthermore, you should express a desire to examine other systems to seek underlying causes of local conditions, eg tell the examiners that you would like to examine the abdomen for secondary causes of hernias or varicose veins.

It is usually up to you whether you talk as you examine or you present your findings at the end. Practise both ways: you may be requested specifically to 'explain what you are doing' or you may be interrupted at any stage of the examination to 'present your findings so far'.

3. An ability to elicit and draw conclusions from physical signs

You will not fail the examination if you do not pick up all the physical signs. However, you will be asked questions such as 'What are the causes of X?' and 'What is the differential diagnosis?' Aim to be one step ahead of your examiners by pre-empting such questions.

Seek clues from the beginning: observe all the artefacts around the patient such as drips and catheters. Plastic gloves next to a patient with a submandibular swelling indicate that you are expected to palpate the gland bimanually. A glass of water next to a patient with a neck swelling suggests a goitre.

Never forget to look at the patient as a whole, even when you are asked to examine one small part: rheumatoid nodules on the elbow suggest the diagnosis before you have even looked at the hands.

OSCEs assess your interpretive skills, preparation and progress, as well as factual recall; they include task-oriented items and they can examine your powers of decision making, problem solving and behavioural attitudes in simulated professional practice. The overall effect is to provide a valid assessment of clinical practice.

4 Frequently asked questions and the viva

Medicine involves a great deal of communication, with both patients and colleagues from all disciplines. Thus presenting clinical findings, answering related questions, and discussing differential diagnoses and subsequent management are a routine part of clinical practice. Do not therefore be surprised to be asked further questions about your clinical findings.

Vivas are widely practised in postgraduate examinations but less so in undergraduate examinations because they can be subjective and provide a patchy assessment of the curriculum. You may particularly dread them because the field is vast and 'they can ask you anything'. The viva does, however, provide an examiner a rapid way of covering essential knowledge in a form that relates to subsequent clinical practice. This is why some schools retain a **pass or fail viva** for borderline candidates.

If you are unfortunate enough to be in this group, take courage from the fact that there are usually two examiners **looking for reasons to pass you**. The examination usually follows a standard approach, and paying attention to the viva techniques outlined below and the content of the subsequent pages will make it less of an ordeal. They are likely to cover a number of topics to ensure that your knowledge across the syllabus is at a safe and competent level for you to progress.

You should also be aware that any part of the clinical examination can turn into a 'mini viva'. The **frequently asked questions** throughout the text cover the topics, and answers, that make up the standard surgical viva.

The other type of viva that you may be fortunate enough to be part of is the **distinction viva** – equally terrifying! Here the rules are different; the examiners are assessing a depth of surgical knowledge beyond the contents of this book. They may start off with the same standard questions, but will then ask the details of probably two topics, pushing you to your limit. You may think that you shouldn't be there and be tempted to withdraw – but don't – it is as an enlightening experience, you can't be marked down and your luck may hold! Scan through topics that have been covered in surgical journals over the last year online and when you find ones that interest you read them in detail – you may have to visit the library to find the full text. The examiners will have read the same material and will enjoy the discussion – good luck.

VIVA TECHNIQUE

Note the following points:

- Go in with a positive attitude.

- Although you will be nervous, try not to show it: aim to give an impression of calm confidence.

- Try to hold the attention of your examiners: speak audibly and clearly. Keep eye contact with at least one of them.

- When asked a question, consider for a moment before rushing into an answer. However, do not hesitate too long because this makes you appear uncertain.

- If you do not understand a question, admit it, put it behind you and be ready for the next question.

- Once you get onto a topic that you know, keep talking as long as you have positive factual knowledge to offer. Drop your voice slightly on the final sentence so that the examiners know that you have completed your statement; try not to peter out.

- Be confident in your knowledge: avoid words such as 'possible' and 'I think'. If an examiner says 'Are you sure?', this does not necessarily mean that you are wrong. If, however, an examiner tells you that you are wrong, accept it, even if you are certain that you are right. This is not the time for argument or confrontation.

- Don't dig yourself a hole by mentioning a very rare condition or something about which you know little or nothing. The examiner could very well ask you to elaborate ('Oh yes, tell me more about that').

- Don't worry if some humour arises and you are excluded: examiners are pleased to have some light relief during a heavy day's examining. However, do not go out of your way to be funny because this can fall very flat.

- At the end, do not rush off as soon as the bell rings: the examiner decides the finishing point, not you. When the end is signalled, smile and thank the examiners, regardless of your feelings. Leave quietly at a normal pace. Try not to trip, knock over the chair or slam the door!

ORGANISATION OF INFORMATION

Always show the examiners that you can classify information. The following 'time-honoured' mnemonics will help you organise your information, but if you make up your own they will be more memorable.

A disease

You may be asked to talk about a particular disease. Use a pathology sieve to structure your answer. One aide-mémoire is 'Dressed In a Surgeon's Gown A Physician Might Make Progress': Definition, Incidence, Sex, Geography, Aetiology, Pathogenesis, Macroscopic pathology, Microscopic pathology, Prognosis. This is modified to form a clinical sieve '… a physician Should Succeed In Treatment': Symptoms, Signs, Investigations, Treatment.

Aetiology

Examiners often ask the causes of a condition. Remember to mention common causes before rarer ones. If you have not memorised a list for that condition, again refer to a sieve. You may find the following mnemonic useful: **CIMETIDINE** – Congenital, Infective, Inflammatory, Metabolic, Endocrine, Traumatic, Iatrogenic, Degenerative, Idiopathic, Neoplastic, Everything else!

An easy surgical specific mnemonic is **TIMEC: T**: tumour/trauma; **I**: infection, inflammation, ischaemia; **M**: mechanical, metabolic; **E**: endocrine; **C**: congenital

Management

The question 'How would you manage a patient with this condition?' comes up again and again. The term 'management' is sometimes used loosely to be synonymous with treatment. However, management refers to history, examination, special investigations *and* treatment. You should *always* begin by saying 'I would take a thorough history and perform a full examination.' Go on to describe the special investigations that you would request and only then describe the treatment. If asked about the management of trauma or shock, never forget to say: 'This is an emergency. I would first check the airway, the breathing and the circulation (ABC).'

Special investigations

When asked about special investigations, start with simple investigations such as urinalysis and blood tests: haematological (FBC, clotting studies, group and save), biochemical (U&Es, LFTs, TFTs, amylase) and urinalysis. Then go on to describe relevant imaging investigations (chest radiograph, ultrasonography and Doppler sonography, angiography, barium studies, CT and MRI), endoscopy and biopsies (cytology and histology). Remember that all older patients being considered for surgery should have a chest radiograph and ECG (think: 1 fluids, 2 tissues and 3 imaging).

Treatment

If asked about the treatment of any disease, always divide your answer into conservative, medical and surgical. Under conservative treatment, consider the contributions from all other healthcare providers such as nurses, physiotherapists, occupational therapists and social services. Under medical treatment, consider drugs, chemotherapy and radiotherapy.

TOPICS COVERED IN OSCES AND VIVAS

Objects used as talking points

Examiners will often have an array of objects in front of them that serve as useful talking points; they may also be incorporated into OSCEs.

Results of investigations

Familiarise yourself with plain radiographs, CT and MRI scans of the skull, chest and abdomen, and barium studies, IVUs and angiograms. Examiners like to know if you have actually seen these investigations and may ask you to describe the procedures. You should also know normal haematological and biochemical values.

Pathology specimens

If handed a pathology pot, look all around the specimen: a discouraging amorphous mass on one view may be easily recognised by the presence of a nipple or an appendix on the other side. Note the organ, describe the abnormalities and make a diagnosis. You may then be asked about the condition and how the patient might have presented.

Other objects

You are expected to recognise a variety of instruments and tubing. These include an endotracheal tube, a laryngoscope, a Guedel airway, a laryngeal mask, a chest drain, a tracheostomy tube, a Sengstaken–Blakemore tube, a T-tube, a proctoscope, sigmoidoscope and an endoscope. You may be asked to describe a practical procedure such as how to catheterise or how to put down an endotracheal tube.

Other popular viva topics

Popular questions are listed at the end of each chapter in this book. You should also be particularly aware of emergencies, anatomy and embryology, and general surgical care.

Emergencies

You must know about the management of the common surgical emergencies such as the acute abdomen and acute upper and lower GI bleeding. These are 'pass/fail' questions.

Anatomy and embryology

You are not expected to know much anatomy, embryology or details of operations. However, there are certain topics that are particularly popular with examiners. These include the anatomy of the appendix, inguinal and femoral canals, tracheostomy sites, and the embryology of thyroglossal and branchial cysts.

General surgical care

It is essential that you know about fluid balance, postoperative complications and complications of fractures, wounds and incisions.

5

The day of the examination

The examination week is very intensive. Each day covers OSLERs/long cases and OSCEs/short cases, and may include a viva. It therefore deserves forethought and preparation, particularly on what you intend to take with you, what you will wear and how you will make your way to the examination.

Take appropriate equipment

Work out in advance exactly what you intend to carry. Know what equipment is in which pocket. Bring the following items:

- Watch with a second hand (carry if bare elbow policy)

- Stethoscope

- Short ruler

- Tape measure

- Pen torch (plus extra batteries)

- Opaque tube, eg an empty Smartie tube (for transillumination)

- Wooden spatulas (for looking in the mouth)

- Tourniquet (for examining varicose veins).

Neurological examination requires additional items that you can bring yourself, although they will usually be provided:

- Cotton wool

- Sterile, sheathed disposable needles (wooden sticks, if against med. school policy)

- Tuning fork

- Tendon hammer

- Orange sticks (for eliciting plantar responses)
- Red- and white-headed hatpins (each >5 mm diameter)
- Pocket-sized reading chart
- Ophthalmoscope.

Dress conventionally

Avoid appearing at all unconventional. Men should wear a plain dark suit, tie and white shirt. Women should wear a smart dress or suit. Hair should be tidy: men should have a recent haircut and women with long hair should tie it back. Make sure that your nails are clean and your shoes polished.

Arrive on time

It is essential that you arrive on time and in a composed state. You can be sure that there will be examiners and patients waiting for you, regardless of traffic delays or train strikes. Excuses wear thin on such occasions. If you are not familiar with the venue, a preliminary visit may be worthwhile in order to time your journey.

Aim to be at the examination at least 30 minutes before the listed starting time. This will ensure that you are able to find the toilets, check your dress and equipment, and fill in any necessary forms. It is a good idea, while waiting outside the examination room, to write down the various headings of your history and examination on the blank paper provided. Not only does this ensure that you do not forget a heading in the heat of the moment, but it limits the space (and hence time) that you spend on any one area.

Section 2
History, examination, typical cases

6

General examination and pain

In surgical finals a long case is usually directed at a single system, and OSCE and short cases at specific clinical signs, as considered in subsequent chapters. Nevertheless be sure that you can undertake a structured general examination that can be integrated with the examination of every system. Pain can be a feature of all systems: be sure that you have a reliable system for questioning – the following can serve as a template, but if you work out your own it will be more memorable.

The History

- Where is the pain? (Ask the patient to point to the area where the pain is felt maximally)
- Have you ever had a pain like this before?
- When did you first notice the pain this time?
- Did the pain begin suddenly or gradually?
- Has the pain become worse since it started?
- Can you describe the pain? (?colicky, ?burning, ?aching)
- How severe is the pain? Does it keep you awake at night?
- Does the pain go anywhere else?
- Is there anything that makes the pain better?
- Is there anything that makes the pain worse?
- What do you think caused the pain?

A mnemonic may help you remember the important features: **S**ite, **R**adiation, **S**everity, **N**ature, **O**nset, **P**eriodicity, **D**uration, **R**elieved by, **A**ccentuated by, **T**iming (eg **S**tate **R**egistered **S**taff **N**urse; **O**ut-**P**atients **D**epartment; **RAT**).

Other common surgical features are lumps, swellings and ulcers (discharge, bleeding), as considered in Chapter 7. In a long case, always quickly survey the past, drug, social, family and systemic histories, as outlined on page 8; if you are short of time, this can be done during the examination, but, as in your future clinical practice, never omit this because unexpected things turn up during this enquiry and the examiner may want to talk about them. Is there a urine sample by the bed that you are expected to test?

THE EXAMINATION

As in all examinations, gain the patient's verbal consent to proceed (see page 8). The general approach assesses the wellbeing of the patient, both the mental and physical conditions; you will already have gained a lot of information during your history taking. The general assessment includes your general impression, and the examination of the hands and the head and neck; this is integrated with the subsequent examination of each system.

ACTION	NOTE
Introduce yourself	
Say what you wish to do	
Ask the patient's permission to proceed	
Stand at the end of the bed and observe the patient	
If the examiner is with you, say what you are looking for (being sensitive to the patient who is listening)	*?does the patient look well, malaise, state of hygiene, are they in pain*
	behaviour, mental status and mood: *?relaxed, cooperative, anxious, apathetic, depressed*
	colour: *?pallor, cyanosed, pigmentation* ±, *breathlessness (if so – respiratory rate)*
	posture, freedom of movement
	weight loss (gain) (increased appetite with loss of weight – *diabetes, thyrotoxicosis, malabsorption*): *starvation, chronic infection, microorganisms, parasites, malignancy*

ACTION	NOTE
	dehydration/oedema
	syndromes: *congenital, endocrine; hepatic and renal failure*
Move to the patient's right side and examine the right hand, followed by the left and compare	hands
	skin of dorsum: *?dry, sweating, thin, thickened, bruising, warts, senile keratosis, nodules, tags, palmar erythema, Dupuytren's contracture*
	rashes: *erythema, macular, papular, vesicular, blisters, scaling, plaques*
	nails: *?bitten, pallor, cyanosis, pitting, leukoplakia, koilonychia, splinter haemorrhages, clubbing*
	joints: *page 154*
	face: *skin, hair, scalp;* conjunctiva – *anaemia;* sclera – *jaundice*
	mouth – gums, teeth: *?caries, ?abnormal mucous membrane, coating, ulcers*
	tremor: fine – *anxiety, thyrotoxicosis;* coarse – *neurological*
	pulse: *rate, rhythm, volume, character, vessel wall*
	blood pressure
	lymphatic enlargement
Proceed to targeted system as considered in subsequent sections	
Cover patient and ensure that they are comfortable	
Organise your findings before presentation	
If examiner is present, turn to him or her and present your findings	

FAQS AND POPULAR VIVA QUESTIONS

1. What are the causes of anaemia?

2. What are the clinical features of anaemia?

3. What are the causes of jaundice?

4. What are the clinical features of jaundice?

5. What are the causes of dehydration?

6. What are the clinical features of dehydration?

7. What are the clinical features of heart failure?

8. What do you understand by Cushing syndrome?

9. What is CPR?

10. What is the emergency management of a patient with major trauma?

ANSWERS

1. **Anaemia** is a decrease in circulating haemoglobin. It can be classified according to the size of the red blood cells (mean corpuscular volume / MCV describes the average volume of a red blood cell):

   a.   Hypochromic microcytic (small size)

   b.   Normochromic normocytic (normal size)

   c.   Macrocytic/megaloblastic (large size).

   Microcytic anaemia is usually linked to iron deficiency:

   a.   Low dietary intake (green vegetables, liver, dairy products)

   b.   Low absorption (increased with acidity)

   c.   Increased iron requirements (usually due to chronic loss – menstrual, gut inflammation and malignancy, worms [hookworm in tropics])

   d.   Chronic disease

   e.   Sideroblastic anaemia.

   Normocytic anaemia is seen in:

   a.   Chronic diseases (liver and renal failure, chronic inflammation and inflammatory bowel disease, drugs, chemicals and malignancy)

   b.   Haemolytic anaemias (sickle, thalassaemia [may also be microcytic], glucose-6-phosphate dehydrogenase deficiency, hereditary spherocytosis)

   c.   Bone marrow disease

   d.   Aplastic anaemia and autoimmune disorders; the anaemia of acute blood loss is delayed until the plasma volume is replaced.

   Megaloblastic anaemia:

   Megaloblasts are formed in the marrow due to defective DNA synthesis; the deficiency is usually of vitamin B_{12} or folic acid. Levels are affected by poor intake, loss of intrinsic factor in the stomach (gastrectomy, gastric atrophy [pernicious anaemia and other autoimmune conditions] alcoholic liver disease and occasionally small-gut and pancreatic disorders.

In surgical patients low haemoglobin (Hb) must alert the surgeon to a **source of blood loss**. This can be:

a. Occult (hidden!), such as slowly bleeding gastric cancer that renders the patient anaemic over a long period of time. The patient may present with fatigue and shortness of breath

b. Acute, as in ruptured oesophageal varices or diverticular disease. The patient may present with haematemesis, melaena or haematochezia (blood per rectum from a lower GI source – not modified as seen in melaena).

Managing 'surgical' anaemias:

A low Hb should prompt the clinician to request an MCV (mean corpuscular volume), iron studies (serum ferritin levels, serum plasma iron and total iron-binding capacity), vitamin B_{12} and folate levels as a baseline set of investigations.

A low Hb with a low MCV and depleted iron levels should prompt further investigation including faecal guaiac testing (looking for occult bleeding in the GI tract) and urine dipstick (blood loss from the renal tract). A full menstrual history needs to be taken in women, as well as an assessment of dietary habits.

The second level of investigation includes a colonoscopy and oesophagoduodenoscopy (OGD) to look for GI pathology.

Failing this, a CT scan of the chest, abdomen and pelvis may be the last resort.

A haematology opinion must always be sought if in doubt regarding the diagnosis.

A CT pneumocolon can be undertaken instead of a colonoscopy in frail patients.

Capsule endoscopy (a small camera that is swallowed by the patient and retrieved when passed in stool) can detect bleeding lesions in the small bowel which cannot be reached with standard endoscopes.

2. Patients are pale but may be asymptomatic, the body compensating by an increased cardiac output and a shift of the oxygen dissociation curve to the right. With progression, there is fatigue, fainting and cardiac signs of shortness of breath, palpitations, angina, claudication and eventually cardiac failure, with signs of tachycardia, a hyperdynamic circulation, a systolic flow murmur and signs of cardiac failure.

   Look for conjunctival pallor; in iron deficiency the nails are brittle and spooned (koilonychia), there may be angular stomatitis, atrophy of tongue papillae and glossitis. Pernicious anaemia may be associated with neurological signs and hepatosplenomegaly, and all anaemias can show the symptoms and signs of an underlying disease. In Plummer–Vinson syndrome, iron deficiency is associated with dysphagia, leading to weight loss.

3. **Jaundice** is the yellow skin discoloration produced by increased levels of circulating bilirubin. This may be due to:

   a. Pre-hepatic: increased production of bilirubin due to increased break-down of red cells (haemolytic anaemias) and congenital hyperbilirubinaemia (Gilbert syndrome being the commonest and mildest form)

   b. Hepatic: obstruction to the normal flow of bilirubin within the liver: this can occur in most forms of acute and chronic liver disease,culminating in end-stage liver failure, which can only be treated by transplantation. Hence, hepatitis and end-stage liver failure in the form of cirrhosis can be mentioned in the exams as a cause of 'hepatic' jaundice. Common causes are viral (hepatitis B/C), alcoholic or autoimmune hepatitis

   c. Post-hepatic (obstruction): obstruction to bilirubin flow after it has left the liver. Post-hepatic obstruction is usually due to gallstones (usually in the presence of right upper quadrant pain), while painless jaundice must raise alarm regarding cancers of the biliary tree and the head of the pancreas. Choledochal cysts are a benign cause of post-hepatic jaundice.

   In the jaundiced patient, measure liver function tests. A high bilirubin confirms the presence of jaundice. NB also check clotting.

Remember that high ALT levels confirm liver injury, while high ALP levels indicate injury to the biliary tree downstream from the liver.

Hence high bilirubin with ALT > ALP suggests a hepatic cause for the jaundice.

A high bilirubin level with ALP > ALT suggests an obstructive cause (post-hepatic) for the jaundice.

To confirm the cause of jaundice request an ultrasound scan. In obstructive jaundice the biliary tree will be dilated as it is obstructed (by a gallstone or tumour). In hepatic jaundice the ultrasound scan will reveal changes in the morphology of the liver parenchyma which would suggest a diagnosis (hepatitis or cirrhosis).

Also remember that in pre-hepatic jaundice the bilirubin is unconjugated (as the liver's metabolic capacity to conjugate is saturated), while in post-hepatic jaundice the bilirubin is conjugated.

4. The symptoms of acute liver disease may be mild, but in viral infections can progress rapidly to malaise, anorexia, fever and unconsciousness. The symptoms of chronic disease depend on the cause; in addition to jaundice there may be pruritus / itching (due to release of conjugated bilirubin, ie not in haemolytic forms) gynaecomastia and testicular atrophy, and as liver failure progresses, abdominal distension from ascites, confusion, drowsiness and bleeding from oesophageal varices; obstructive disease can manifest as pale stools as well as dark urine. Biliary symptoms include indigestion, colic and fever; pancreatic pain occurs in the upper abdomen and radiates through to the back.

    On examination:

    a. Early jaundice is first observed in the frenulum of the tongue and best observed in the sclera of the eyes, progressing to widespread cutaneous staining

    b. Look for xanthomas around the eyes; in the hands look for palmar erythema, spider naevi, clubbing and Dupuytren's contracture (most often in alcoholic cirrhosis); in later stages liver flap (of the wrist), altered consciousness and generalised purpura

c. in the abdomen the patient develops collateral veins around the umbilicus (caput medusa), hepatosplenomegaly (the liver may shrink in late stages of cirrhosis; splenic enlargement usually indicates portal hypertension); palpable gallbladder (Courvoisier said it was unlikely to be a stone!); ascites (make sure you percuss for it); abdominal masses (look for associated disease, such as colonic cancer and lymphomas).

Remember that the symptoms and signs in liver failure are caused by portal hypertension or impaired synthetic function of the liver.

Portal hypertension (as blood flow through the liver is impaired due to structural changes brought about by cirrhosis). This causes splenomegaly (as drainage of splenic blood is obstructed) and collateral blood routes form at the site of porto-systemic anastomoses. These give rise to oesophageal and haemorrhoidal varices, as well as a caput medusa

Impaired synthetic function of the liver:

a. High oestrogen: increased systemic vascularity (spider naevi), gynaecomastia, testicular atrophy

b. Low albumin: ascites

c. Poor synthesis of clotting function causing coagulopathies, bleeding and bruising

d. Encephalopathy: an impairment of brain function due to ineffective metabolism of ammonia

e. Impaired bilirubin metabolism, giving rise to jaundice.

5. **Dehydration** is caused by reduced intake or excessive loss of fluid. Also consider electrolyte balance, whether the tissues are hyper-, hypo- or isotonic: in most situations it is isotonic and replacement is with isotonic fluids. Dehydration is a particular problem in neonates and in the elderly. Lack of intake occurs in the unconscious patient; an inability to swallow; malnutrition; fasting; pre- and postoperative deprivation; lack of water at sea (sea water rapidly produces a hypertonic state that progresses to renal failure).

Losses are usually due to vomiting and diarrhoea (cholera causing extreme loss but other infections can also be rapidly lethal); fistulae; burns; major trauma and blood loss. Fluid may be sequestrated, as in paralytic ileus. Excess sweating and hyperthermia usually occur in hot countries but can result from prolonged exercise without adequate fluids (eg marathon, triathlon). People in protective clothing (eg chemical protection) are more liable to dehydration and hyperthermia in hot climates. Polyuria is a complication of diabetes insipidus, diabetes mellitus, hypercalcaemia, some uraemic states, diuretics and postoperatively – all requiring measured fluid and electrolyte balance and avoidance of over-zealous uncontrolled replacement.

6. Early symptoms of dehydration are thirst and a reduced and concentrated urine output. There may be nausea, vomiting, cramps, weakness, paraesthesia and orthostatic hypotension (a drop in blood pressure when standing). Cerebral symptoms of a reduced circulating volume include headache, 'hangover' sensation, dizziness and fainting, progressing to delirium, seizures and unconsciousness.

   Signs include tachycardia, hypotension and pyrexia. The skin is dry and lax (check over the back of the hands); dry tongue; dry or cracked lips; sunken eyes with absent lacrimation. Altered mental state is present as symptoms progress.

7. **Cardiac failure** occurs when the cardiac output is insufficient to meet the metabolic and perfusion needs of the body. It may be due to damage to the heart muscle, its valves or the conduction system, or to abnormal filling, and is variously classified by the cause, severity and the side of the heart most affected.

   Anatomical classification of causes of cardiac failure (external to internal):

   a. Pericardium: pericardial effusion, pericarditis

   b. Myocardium: ischemia (myocardial infarct), cardiomyopathy

   c. Endocardium: valvular problems (stenosis or regurgitation)

   d. Electrical: arrhythmias

   e. Pre- or post-cardiac vascular: fluid overload, hypertension, pulmonary embolism, aortic dissection.

Heart failure can arise from the right heart, the left heart or (eventually) both sides.

In heart failure blood 'accumulates' in the vascular territory preceding the failing chamber: the lungs (left heart failure) and the systemic venous circulation (right heart failure).

Left heart failure causes congestion (build-up) of blood on the lungs. This gives rise to fluid exudation in the lungs and pulmonary oedema (so tachypnoea, shortness of breath, low oxygen saturation, impaired gas exchange on an ABG and bilateral widespread crackles).

Right-sided heart failure causes a raised central venous pressure in the major veins of the body (so raised central venous pressure / JVP).

SVC congestion: raised JVP.

IVC congestion: hepatomegaly, peripheral oedema.

In reality this is a simplistic model and clinical signs may overlap. More typical heart failure can present with a combination of palpitations, fatigue, syncope, cough, shortness of breath, respiratory crackles, frothy sputum, orthopnoea, paroxysmal nocturnal dyspnoea and angina.

Cardiac signs of heart failure include altered pulse rate, rhythm, volume and character, abnormal blood pressure, cardiomegaly and abnormal heart sounds; in the hands look for clubbing and cyanosis. Fluid retention presents with pulmonary added sounds, pleural effusion, peripheral oedema, ascites, raised jugular venous pressure, hepatomegaly and a hepatojugular reflex. Additional signs include those of high-output conditions – anaemia, thyrotoxicosis, arteriovenous fistulae and malformations, Paget's disease, beri beri and septicaemia.

Cor pulmonale is a right-sided heart failure caused by lung pathology, eg pulmonary hypertension secondary to recurrent pulmonary emboli.

8. **Cushing syndrome** is caused by an excess of free circulating glucocorticoids. Its aetiology can be classified as:

   a. Exogenous steroids: due to steroid therapy for other medical condition (commonest cause); eg oral steroids following organ transplantation

   b. Increased ACTH production in the pituitary gland, eg pituitary hyperplasia or ACTH-secreting pituitary adenomas (Cushing's disease)

   c. Increased steroid production in the adrenal glands, eg adrenal hyperplasia, adenoma, adenocarcinoma

   d. Ectopic sources: ACTH-producing tumours, eg small-cell carcinoma of the lung.

Cushing syndrome may be complicated by problems of hypertension, diabetes mellitus, polyuria, peptic ulcer, pancreatitis, susceptibility to infection, impotence, amenorrhoea, infertility, hypercalcaemia, osteoporosis, muscle weakness, sleep deprivation and psychological disturbances. Excess ACTH secretion can also be accompanied by hyperkalaemia and hyperpigmentation.

The clinical signs of moon face, facial acne and a buffalo hump are diagnostic. The skin is thin with telangectasia, purpuric patches, purple abdominal stretch marks and hyperhidrosis. The hair is dry and brittle and of male distribution, often with baldness. Suprasellar extension of pituitary lesions may compress the optic chiasm, with resultant bi-temporal hemianopia.

9. **Cardiopulmonary resuscitation** is an emergency procedure for the treatment of cardiac arrest. It involves rhythmical compression on the chest to maintain pulmonary and systemic blood flow, combined with exhalation into the patient's mouth, or other means of artificial ventilation, to inflate the lungs and maintain end-organ perfusion and oxygen delivery.

Guidelines vary, but a useful regimen is to apply 30 compressions at 100–120 beats/min, at a depth of a third of the chest (5–6 cm): alternated with 2 rescue breaths. For effective rescue breaths, create a seal around the mouth, squeeze the nose and exhale for 1 second, checking for the rise and fall of the chest. Although CPR is only effective in about 10% of cases, it can delay tissue death until more advanced life support (intravenous drugs and defibrillation) becomes available. Successful CPR depends on resuscitation technique, underlying cause of the cardiac arrest and the patient's physiological reserve.

10. The resuscitation of the trauma patient must be undertaken according to **ATLS guidelines** (Advanced Trauma Life Support) produced by the American College of Surgeons. All doctors involved in trauma care should gain this qualification. The following provides a brief summary for finals purposes:

Check for danger to yourself or the patient.

Check for patient response (do they respond if you firmly shake their shoulders and ask them to open their eyes if they can hear you: shake and shout)

Shout for help / put out the hospital trauma call via switchboard.

AIRWAY and C-Spine immobilisation –

1. If there is any suggestion of neck injury, immobilise the cervical spine using a collar and blocks.

2. Open their **A**irway by performing a head-tilt / chin-lift procedure. Use airway adjuncts such as Guedel airway or a nasopharyngeal airway if basic manoeuvres fail. Administer oxygen (100% via a face mask). Advanced airway manoeuvres involve endotracheal intubation or the use of a LMA (laryngeal mask airway).

BREATHING – Check for **B**reathing by holding your ear close to their mouth, listening and feeling for their breath on your cheek and looking for the rise and fall of their chest. Check oxygen saturation. Look for evidence of haemothorax, pneumothorax, flail chest or mediastinal injury (cardiac tamponade, traumatic aortic dissection). Haemo / pneumothoraces require insertion of a chest drain. Tension pneumothorax requires initial decompression with a large-bore cannula in the second intercostal space, midclavicular line. Pericardial tamponade requires needle pericardiocentesis (aspiration). Major vessel or mediastinal trauma requires thoracotomy or sternotomy. Further tests: ABG – perform an arterial blood gas to check the patient's gas exchange (pH, pCO_2, pO_2). Are they in respiratory failure?

CIRCULATION – Check for presence of Circulation. Feel a central pulse (carotid or femoral) – if absent commence CPR and follow the Advanced Life Support (ALS) algorhythm. Advanced circulation assessment involves checking heart rate, blood pressure, JVP, heart sounds, peripheral perfusion (warmth and capillary refill time in the toes). If there is any evidence of external bleeding stop this by simple manual compression. Insert two large intravenous cannulae and administer fluid or blood products if the patient is in hypovolaemic shock. Fluid resuscitation is a much debated subject. In trauma victims, warm fluid should be used to avoid hypothermia. Overly aggressive fluid therapy may cause already formed clots in injured vessels to be displaced, having an overall detrimental effect. Further tests: ECG. Attach to cardiac monitor.

If the patient has obvious major bleeding that will be worsened by CPR, put pressure on the wound and elevate the limb that is damaged before commencing the above algorithm. Lay the patient down if possible, and dress the wound(s) with a maximum of two bandages. If blood seeps through, remove the bandages and start again.

DISABILITY – Check body temperature and glucose levels. Check for any evidence of neurological injury: GCS (Glasgow coma scale), pupil size, reaction and accommodation, gross motor and sensory function of upper and lower limbs. Further tests: CT scan of the head.

EVERYTHING ELSE: Abdomen.

Look for any obvious wounds or bruising indicating penetrating and blunt injury respectively. Palpate for right upper quadrant pain or masses (liver injury / haematoma) and left upper quadrant pain (splenic injury / haematoma).

Palpate the pelvis for any evidence of instability or pain suggestive of pelvic fracture (this can cause major internal bleeding by injuring the iliac vessels).

Look at the penile meatus in men for blood, suggestive of urethral injury (contraindication for Foley catheterisation).

Perform a log-roll to inspect for injuries to the back and spine; at this time do a digital rectal examination to assess anal sphincter tone or presence of lower GI bleeding.

Further tests: **F**AST scan (focused assessment with sonography for trauma). This is an abdominal and thoracic ultrasound assessment looking for evidence of free fluid in the abdomen and chest. Presence of fluid would mandate urgent operative intervention in **unstable** patients not fit to undergo formal imaging with a CT scan.

Take a short, focused trauma history using the **AMPLE** mnemonic:

A: any **allergies**?

M: do you take any **medicines** (drug history)?

P: any **past medical problems** / history?

L: when did you **last eat** (to assess risk of intubation / rapid sequence induction of anaesthesia should it be needed)?

E: events – how did the injury happen?

At the end perform a trauma series of X-rays: C-spine, chest and pelvis. Further imaging is requested once the patient has completed the primary survey.

Ideally each component of the primary survey should be performed by different individuals feeding back to the trauma lead, so that the initial assessment should not last more than a few minutes.

If the patient is stable, proceed to a formal, detailed assessment, the secondary survey.

7 Swellings and ulcers

THE HISTORY

Swellings and ulcers are presenting features of many diseases. Always ask the same questions.

- When did you first notice it?

- How did you notice it?

- Has it changed since you first noticed it?

- Has it ever completely disappeared since you noticed it?

- How does it bother you? (What are the main symptoms: is it painful or tender?)

- Do you have (or have you ever had) any other lumps or ulcers?

- What do you think caused it?

THE EXAMINATION

Even if the diagnosis seems obvious, always go through the same routine when examining a swelling or an ulcer. It is probably easier to talk as you go rather than to present your findings at the end.

'Examine this patient's swelling'

ACTION	NOTE
Introduce yourself	
Say what you wish to do	
Ask the patient's permission to proceed	
Expose the lump completely	
LOOK	
Inspect the lump	*?shape*
	?colour
Measure:	
• distance from the nearest bony prominence	*?position*
• dimensions	*?size*
FEEL	
Ask if the lump is tender/painful	Note if any part is sensitive on subsequent palpation
a. Temperature	
Run the backs of your fingers over the surface and surrounding area	*?warm*
b. Surface	
Feel with the pulps of your fingers	*?smooth*
	?bosselated
	?rough
c. Edge	
Feel with your finger and thumb	*?clearly/poorly defined*
d. Consistency	*?stony-hard, ?rubbery hard*
	?spongy, ?soft

ACTION	NOTE
e. Surrounding area	*?indurated*
	?invaded
	?colour change
PRESS	
a. Pulsatility	
Rest a finger of each hand on opposite sides of the lump for a few seconds	*?expansile pulsation* (fingers pushed apart)
Watch your fingers	*?transmitted pulsation* (fingers pushed in same direction)
b. Compressibility/reducibility	
Press the lump firmly and then release the pressure	*?compressible* (lump disappears on pressure and reappears on release)
	?reducible (lump reappears only on application of another force, eg coughing, gravity)
c. Percussion	
Percuss over lump	*?dull*
	?resonant
d. Fluctuation/fluid thrill	
Place two fingers of one hand at opposite ends of the lump	Use this test for a *small* lump
Press the middle of the lump with the index finger of your other hand	*?fluctuant* (two fingers move apart when middle area pressed)
Repeat in a perpendicular plane	
Ask patient to place the edge of his or her hand in the middle of the swelling	Use this test for a *large* swelling
Flick on one side and feel on other side for a percussion wave	*?fluid thrill*

ACTION	NOTE
MOVE	
Try to move the skin over the lump	*?fixation to skin* (skin cannot be moved over lump)
Try to move the lump in two planes at right angles to each other	*?mobility*
Ask patient to tense the underlying muscle	*?attachment to underlying muscle* (movement *reduced* when underlying muscle tensed or 'disappears' beneath it)
Reassess mobility	
LISTEN	
Auscultate over the lump	*?bruit*
	?bowel sounds
TRANSILLUMINATE	
Press a pen torch and an opaque tube (eg a Smartie tube) on opposite sides of the lump	*?transilluminable* (transillumination can only be accurately assessed by looking down the opaque tube)
Look down the opaque tube	
EXAMINE SURROUNDING TISSUES	
Examine regional lymph nodes:	*?local lymphadenopathy*
• limbs/trunk – axillary nodes	
• head/neck – cervical nodes	
Test sensation in the surrounding area	*?local neurological deficit*
Test the power of related muscles	*?weakness*

'Examine this patient's ulcer'

ACTION	NOTE
Introduce yourself	
Say what you wish to do	
Ask the patient's permission to proceed	
LOOK	
Measure:	
• distance from the nearest bony prominence	*?position*
• dimensions	*?size*
	?shape
Measure the depth in mm	*?depth*
Inspect the base and its coverings	colour: *?red/granulation tissue*
	penetration: *?tendon*
	?bone
	discharge: *?blood*
	?fistula
	?pus
Inspect the edge	edge: *?flat sloping:*

?punched out:

ACTION	NOTE
	?raised:
	?raised and everted:
FEEL	
Ask if the surrounding area is tender	
Feel with the backs of your fingers	*?warm*
EXAMINE SURROUNDING TISSUES	
Examine the regional lymph nodes	*?local lymphadenopathy*
Test sensation in the surrounding area	*?local neurological deficit*
Test the power of related muscles	
Note pulses	

TYPICAL CASES

1. LUMPS AND SWELLINGS

Neck, breast, abdomen and knee swellings are covered on pages 58–81, 82–95, 96–123, and 182–184. This section revises skin lumps, giving examples of common short cases.

Lesions derived from the epidermis

Case 1: squamous cell papilloma/skin tag

This is a pedunculated overgrowth of skin. It is soft, the colour of normal skin and can occur at any site.

Treatment: excision if symptomatic or cosmetic concerns, tying base where possible.

Case 2: wart

Warts are grey/brown filiform lesions, usually seen on the back of the hand. The surface is rough and the consistency hard.

Treatment: if symptoms, paint with podophyllin, freeze or curettage.

Case 3: seborrhoeic keratosis/senile wart

These are flattened, well-defined plaques, usually found on the back. They may be multiple and are usually pigmented. The patient will probably be elderly. They are easily recognised because of their greasy, rough surface and because they are easy to pick off (although you should not try to do this if you are uncertain of the diagnosis).

Case 4: pigmented naevus or malignant melanoma

Benign naevi may occur anywhere. They may be flat, raised, hairy or non-hairy. The surface may be rough or smooth.

You should know the characteristics that suggest malignancy:

- Increase in size
- Ulceration
- Change in colour
- Irritation
- Bleeding
- Halo of pigmentation
- Satellite nodules
- Enlarged local lymph nodes
- Evidence of distant spread.

Treatment: excision biopsy of all suspicious lesions, insuring adequate wide excision margins are taken pending formal diagnosis. Confirmed malignant melanomas require formal staging, wide local excision of affected lesion and relevant lymph nodes as well as chemoradiotherapy.

Note: squamous cell and basal cell carcinomas can also present as epidermal nodules. They usually ulcerate and are considered on page 55.

Lesions derived from the dermis

Case 5: dermatofibroma/histiocytoma

This is a firm nodule, usually seen on the lower leg, containing lipid-filled macrophages. It is part of the skin and fully mobile.

Treatment: excise if symptoms.

Case 6: pyogenic granuloma

This is a bright-red or blood-encrusted nodule. It feels fleshy and is slightly compressible. It bleeds easily.

If you are not sure of the diagnosis, ask the patient how quickly it appeared (it arises within days) and whether he or she remembers a preceding penetrating injury.

Note: unlike the implication of its name, it is not granulomatous or pyogenic. It is actually an acquired haemangioma.

Treatment: excision.

Case 7: keloid scar or hypertrophic scars

Keloid is an overgrowth of fibrous tissue within a scar. Suspect this in an Afro-Caribbean patient who has had recent surgery.

You may be asked about the differences between a keloid and a hypertrophic scar.

	Hypertrophic scar	Keloid scar
Overall incidence	More common	Less common
Association with race?	No	Yes: more common in African–Caribbean people
Extent of overgrowth	Confined to scar tissue	Extends into surrounding tissue
Resolves spontaneously?	Yes: within a few months	No
Recurs after surgery?	No	Yes

Treatment:

1. Compression therapy or occlusive dressing

2. Injection of steroids in lesion

3. Topical agents: vitamin E, steroid creams

4. Surgical excision is associated with recurrence. If ablation is needed cryotherapy, laser or radiotherapy may be attempted.

Lesions derived from skin appendages

Case 8: keratoacanthoma/molluscum sebaceum

A keratoacanthoma is a benign overgrowth of a sebaceous gland.

It appears within 3–4 weeks. It resembles a volcano, consisting of a conical lump of normal skin colour with a central irregular crater containing keratin.

It usually regresses spontaneously but may take 6–9 months.

Treatment: excise only if diagnosis is uncertain or marked symptoms.

Case 9: keratin horn

This is a dry, hard spike, derived from sebaceous secretions. Unlike a keratoacanthoma, it does not regress.

Treatment: excise if symptoms.

Case 10: sebaceous cyst

This is an extremely common short case. It is usually found in hairy areas (the scalp, neck, face and scrotum).

The size varies but the lump is usually hemispherical with a well-defined edge. Although it lies subcutaneously, it is attached to skin by the sebaceous duct, hence the skin over it cannot be 'pinched'/elevated.

The *consistency* is hard although there is some fluctuation. It is not usually transilluminable.

Always look for a punctum: only 50% will possess one but it is pathognomonic if found.

If the cyst is painful and red, this does not necessarily indicate infection: after trauma, the secretions may cause a foreign body inflammatory response in the surrounding tissues. Bacteria cannot, however, usually be cultured.

If you are asked about its origin, remember that the term 'sebaceous' cyst is a misnomer. It is **not** derived from the sebaceous gland, but from the outer sheath of the hair follicle. The cyst contents, although thick and waxy, are dead epithelial elements rather than sebaceous secretions.

Treatment:

1.   Antibiotics for cellulitis

2.   Incision and drainage if cyst becomes infected

3.   Elective complete excision of cyst in the absence of infection, followed by primary closure.

Case 11: boil or carbuncle

A boil or furuncle is an infection originating in a hair follicle. It begins as a hard, red, tender lesion. It later discharges spontaneously.

If you are allowed to ask the patient a few questions, ask about diabetes, steroid therapy and other predisposing immunodeficiencies.

You may be asked to describe the differences between a furuncle and a carbuncle.

	Furuncle	Carbuncle
Site	Skin	Subcutaneous tissue
Number of abscesses seen	One	Several
Appearance	Discrete lesion	Generalised necrotic area

Treatment: wait for resolution unless cellulitis is present (antibiotic) or abscess (drain).

Case 12: hydradenitis suppurativa

A red, tender swelling is not necessarily a boil: if the patient has *multiple* such lesions in the *axillae* or *groin*, suspect hydradenitis suppurativa. This is a recurrent infection of sweat (apocrine) glands characterised by subcutaneous sinus and fistula formation.

Treatment:

1.   Antibiotics for early lesions

2.   Incision and drainage of localised abscesses

3. Long-term antibiotics with systemic steroids may be needed for chronic lesions

4. Oral retinoids may be of benefit, but side-effect profile needs to be considered

5. Wide excision of recurrent lesions, with skin flaps or grafts for closure of large defects.

Lesions derived from vascular structures

The term 'haemangioma' encompasses many lesions, including Campbell de Morgan spots and spider naevi.

You should also be able to recognise the two common paediatric haemangiomas.

Case 13: strawberry naevus

This is a bright-red, strawberry-like lesion. It is small at birth but increases in size and may be disfiguring.

Treatment: it should be left alone, because it spontaneously regresses by the age of about 4–5 years. Remember the important exception to this rule is when it obscures a visual field.

Case 14: port-wine stain

This is a flat purple/red lesion with an irregular border and is caused by a capillary malformation of the dermis. It is present at birth and does not increase or decrease in size thereafter. Facial haemangiomas may develop in the distribution of a sensory dermatome. They may be associated with a meningeal haemangioma (Sturge-Weber syndrome).

Treatment: cosmetic creams or tattooing (although not routine). Pulse-dye laser (PDL) therapy may be of benefit.

Lesions not attached to skin

Case 15: lipoma

This is a benign tumour of adipocytes. Its size varies. The *shape* is hemispherical and the *edge* is well defined. The *consistency* is soft and the *surface* bosselated. The overlying skin is easily elevated.

Note: only **large** lipomas are fluctuant and transilluminable.

Lipomas are usually freely mobile although they may occasionally lie beneath the deep fascia.

Treatment: excision.

Case 16: dermoid cyst

Dermoid cysts are hard and spherical. Although derived from epithelial elements within the dermis, they lie subcutaneously.

In an adult, you should suspect an *implantation* dermoid, usually found on the fingers. Ask about a preceding injury.

In a child, suspect a *congenital* dermoid. This occurs at the sites of fusion of the facial processes, eg the outer angle of the eye.

Treatment: excision of whole lesion with primary closure. Prior ultrasound imaging may be needed in certain lipomas to ensure these don't extend deep to muscular planes.

Case 17: ganglion

The patient will have a smooth, hemispherical swelling near a joint or tendon. The most common sites are at the wrist, on the dorsum of the hand and around the ankle. The *surface* is smooth and the *consistency* firm. It is slightly fluctuant and weakly transilluminable.

Remember to palpate the ganglion in all positions of the underlying joint: its mobility depends on whether it is derived from, and thus attached to, deep structures.

Note that the origin is controversial. Some view it as a pocket of synovium, communicating with the associated joint. Others see it as a myxomatous degeneration of fibrous tissue, derived from the tendon sheath.

Treatment: excision. Remember 'hitting with Bible' – the examiners will, but not to be recommended.

2. ULCERS

You should know the definition of an ulcer: a defect in an epithelial surface. You may be asked the causes.

Type	Cause	Underlying disease
Venous (page 229) (75% of leg ulcers)	(1) Superficial venous insufficiency	• Varicose veins
	(2) Deep venous insufficiency	• Previous DVT
Arterial (page 217)	(1) Large-vessel disease (ischaemic)	• Atheroma • Buerger's disease
	(2) Small-vessel disease (vasculitis)	• Rheumatoid arthritis • Polyarteritis nodosa
Traumatic	(1) Neuropathic/ trophic	• Alcohol • Diabetes mellitus • Tabes dorsalis • Syringomyelia
	(2) Others	• Bedsores • Self-inflicted injury
Infective	Often associated with malnutrition	• Pyogenic organisms • Tertiary syphilis • *Mycobacterium ulcerans* • Tropical
Neoplastic	(1) Primary neoplasm	• Squamous cell carcinoma • Basal cell carcinoma • Malignant melanoma
	(2) Secondary neoplasm	

Case 18: ulcer with a sloping edge

A sloping edge is characteristic of a *healing* ulcer, ie a *traumatic* (although not neuropathic) ulcer or a *venous* ulcer.

Venous ulcers are found in the 'gaiter area' (above the malleoli, particularly the medial malleolus). They are usually shallow and flat. The base is covered with pink granulation tissue mixed with white fibrous tissue.

Look for and describe associated signs of superficial or deep venous insufficiency (see page 229).

Case 19: ulcer with a 'punched-out' edge

It is unlikely that you will see a gumma of tertiary syphilis, which is the classic 'punched-out' ulcer. This usually occurs on the anterior aspect of the lower leg and is easily recognised by the yellow-coloured ('wash-leather') base. Ischaemic and neuropathic ulcers are much more common as short cases. They have many of the same characteristics:

- Over the tips of and between the toes

- Over pressure areas (heel, malleoli)

- Pale-pink base (very little granulation tissue)

- Deeply penetrating

- Bone, ligaments and tendons seen in the base.

Ischaemic ulcers are secondary to circulatory insufficiency (large- or small- vessel disease) whereas *neuropathic ulcers* are usually secondary to spinal cord disease or a peripheral neuropathy: repeated injury arises from loss of pain. Remember that in diabetes mellitus ulcers have a *mixed* pathogenesis (see page 217).

If you are asked to distinguish between the two, use the scheme in the table opposite.

	Ischaemic ulcer	Neuropathic ulcer
Ask if the ulcer is painful	Painful	Painless
Look for associated black eschar	Present	Absent
Feel the temperature of the surrounding area	Cold	Warm
Test the sensation of the surrounding area	Sensation intact	Sensation lost

Case 20: ulcer with a raised edge

Ulcers with raised edges are neoplastic. The centre of the carcinoma becomes necrotic, but the periphery continues to grow and rises above the surface of the surrounding skin.

The main features distinguishing a basal cell carcinoma (rodent ulcer) from a squamous cell carcinoma are the *edge* and the *colour*.

	Basal cell carcinoma (BCC)	Squamous cell carcinoma (SCC)
Edge	Raised (smooth)	Raised and everted (irregular)
Colour	Pearly, glistening, pink tinge (due to fine telangiectasia)	Red–brown (due to vascularity)

You should be able to list the predisposing factors for skin cancer:

- Age
- Sunlight (ultraviolet radiation)
- Ionising radiation
- Chemical irritants (eg soot, dyes, tar).

Remember that malignant change (usually to squamous cell carcinoma) can also occur in long-standing benign ulcers (Marjolin's ulcers), in scars and in chronically discharging osteomyelitis sinuses.

Treatment of ulcers:

- Venous – four-layer compression bandaging

- Neuropathic – daily inspection of feet, protect against trauma, clean and bandage

- Arterial – improve blood supply by revascularisation or angioplasty, debridement; amputation if it becomes a source of sepsis or if causing reduced quality of life / mobility when healing is unlikely despite maximum revascularisation attempts

- Infective – treat cause, antibiotics for cellulitis, drain abscesses

- Malignant – excise lesion together with draining lymph nodes; chemotherapy and radiotherapy as adjunctive or palliative options

- Non-malignant – skin graft for persistent ulcers once base granulated.

FAQS AND POPULAR VIVA QUESTIONS

1. Describe the features you would note in examining a lump/an ulcer. How would these features help in your differential diagnosis?

2. What is the difference between a furuncle and a carbuncle?

3. What are the differences between a keloid and a hypertrophic scar?

4. What are the features that would suggest malignancy in a pigmented naevus?

5. Describe the differences in appearance between a basal cell carcinoma and a squamous cell carcinoma.

6. What aetiological factors can predispose to squamous cell carcinoma?

ANSWERS

1. See examination section pages 41–45.

2. A boil is an abscess in a superficial hair follicle. In a carbuncle, the infection has extended into the subcutaneous tissue and it may be a collection of subcutaneous abscesses with or without external tracts.

3. A hypertrophic scar resolves within 6 months. Keloids extend into the surrounding tissues and recur after surgery. One or more steroid injections may help. Keloids are more common in African–Caribbean people.

4. Itching, colour change, increase in size, ulceration, bleeding, halo of pigmentation, satellite nodules, enlarged local lymph nodes and distant spread.

5. Basal cell carcinoma has a smooth, rounded, pink, pearly edge; squamous cell carcinoma has an irregular, raised, everted, red–brown edge.

6. Age, sunlight, ionising radiation and chemicals such as soot, dyes and tar.

Neck swellings and thyroid lumps

THE HISTORY

If your patient complains of a swelling in the neck, ask the same questions as for any lump (page 40).

If you suspect **lymphadenopathy**, ask the following questions to determine local causes:

- Do you have any mouth ulcers or pain in your mouth?

- Do you have any pain or discharge from your nose or ears? Do you have a sore throat?

- Have you noticed any other lumps on your head or face? Do you have any difficulty swallowing?

- Do you have any difficulty breathing?

Your systemic enquiry will be important in determining *generalised* causes. If you suspect a **goitre**, ask the following specific questions.

Local effects of the swelling

- Is the lump painful?

- Do you have any difficulty or pain when you swallow?

- Do you have any difficulty breathing?

- Have you noticed any change in your voice recently?

Eye problems associated with hyperthyroidism

- Do you have double vision?

- Do you get painful, red eyes?

Systemic enquiry to determine thyroid status

1. General symptoms

- Have you noticed a change in your appearance?

- Are you intolerant of hot or cold temperatures?

2. Gastrointestinal symptoms

- Have you noticed a change in your appetite/weight/bowel habit?

3. Cardiorespiratory symptoms

- Do you get palpitations/shortness of breath on exertion/ankle swelling/chest pain?

4. Neurological symptoms

- Have you noticed any nervousness/irritability/insomnia/loss of concentration?

5. Gynaecological symptoms (in females)

- Have you noticed any change in your menstrual cycle?

THE EXAMINATION

A common instruction in the short case is to 'examine this patient's neck' without being given any clue as to the pathology. Alternatively, you may be asked to 'examine this patient's thyroid gland'. In this case, proceed to the relevant section of the examination scheme below. Rarely, you may be pointed out a lump and asked to describe it (pages 40–43).

The presence of a glass of water near the patient is a good hint that there may be a goitre!

Always describe the position of neck swellings in terms of the triangles of the neck.

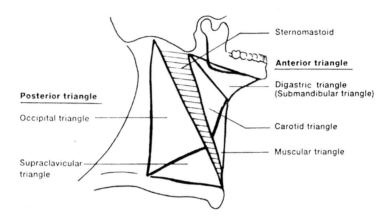

Sternomastoid

Anterior triangle

Digastric triangle
(Submandibular triangle)

Posterior triangle

Occipital triangle

Carotid triangle

Muscular triangle

Supraclavicular
triangle

'Examine this patient's neck'

ACTION	NOTE
Introduce yourself	
Say what you wish to do	
Ask the patient's permission to proceed	
Expose the neck, with the patient sitting up comfortably	
LOOK	
Observe from in front and from either side	*?hyperaemia of skin*
	?scars
	?distended neck veins
	?obvious goitre (between thyroid cartilage and manubrium sterni)
Ask patient to take a sip of water and to hold it in his or her mouth	
Then ask patient to swallow	*?goitre* (moves on swallowing)
Ask patient to stick out tongue	*?thyroglossal cyst* (moves up when tongue stuck out)

Now proceed as follows:

- If *obvious goitre*, continue examination of thyroid gland: A (below)

- If *no goitre*, examine for cervical lymphadenopathy: B (page 64)

- If you *feel an obvious lump*, proceed to C (page 65)

- If you *suspect enlargement of a salivary gland*, proceed to D (page 66)

A. Examination of the thyroid gland

ACTION	NOTE
Introduce yourself	
Say what you wish to do	
Ask the patient's permission to proceed	
LOOK (see previous page)	
FEEL	
Stand behind patient	
Ask if the swelling is tender	
Feel with the flat of your fingers over the thyroid (thumbs posteriorly)	
Tell patient to take another sip of water, to hold it in his or her mouth and then to swallow	*?thyroid felt to move on swallowing*
Palpate gently	*?tender*
	?diffusely enlarged swelling
	?single nodule
	?multinodular goitre
	?texture
	?surface

ACTION	NOTE
	?*approximate size*
Palpate the cervical lymph nodes	?*associated lymphadenopathy* (page 64)
While still standing behind patient, look over the top of his or her head	?*exophthalmos*
ASSESS POSITION	
Stand in front of patient	
Palpate the trachea in the suprasternal notch	?*trachea deviated*
Push each lobe to the opposite side to emphasise contralateral features	?*any previously unnoted features*
Percuss the thyroid	?*lower limit of retrosternal extension*
Auscultate over the thyroid	?*bruit*
ASSESS THYROID FUNCTION	
a. Observe overall	
Look at patient's:	
• face and skin	?*dry/shiny skin*
• build	?*thin/fat*
• dress	?*appropriate for temperature*
• behaviour	?*agitated/lethargic*
b. Examine the hands	
Look at:	
• palms	?*palmar erythema*
• nails	?*thyroid acropachy*
Feel:	
• palms	?*sweaty*

ACTION	NOTE
• pulse	*?tachycardia*
	?large volume
	?atrial fibrillation
Ask patient to hold arms outstretched (exaggerated by placing sheet of paper on them)	*?fast postural tremor*
c. Examine the eyes	
Look at:	
• conjunctiva	*?chemosis/oedema/redness*
• relationship of eyelid to iris	*?lid retraction*
Ask patient to follow your finger up and down	*?lid lag*
Test the eye movements:	
• Ask patient to follow a white hatpin with their eyes	*?ophthalmoplegia*
• Ask him or her to report any double vision	
d. Assess neurologically	
Ask patient to rise from a squatting position (or chair) without using hands for support	*?proximal myopathy* (a sensitive indicator of hypo-/hyperthyroidism)
Test reflexes, observing the relaxation phase:	*?slow-relaxing reflexes* (suggests hypothyroidism)
• supinator	
• biceps	

B. Examination for cervical lymphadenopathy

ACTION	NOTE
Introduce yourself	
Say what you wish to do	
Ask the patient's permission to proceed	
Stand behind patient	
Examine lymph nodes *systematically:*	
First feel the horizontal ring around the skull base:	
• submental	
• submandibular	
• preauricular	
• postauricular	
• occipital	
Then feel the vertical chain:	*?position of enlarged nodes*
• deep cervical	
• posterior triangle	
• supraclavicular	
If you feel enlarged cervical lymph nodes:	
Look in the mouth, ears and throat with pen torch	*?primary site of infection*
	?primary malignancy
Say that you would request a full ENT examination	
Look carefully at the face and all over the scalp	

ACTION	NOTE
Examine: • inguinal nodes • axillary nodes • epitrochlear nodes	*?generalised lymphadenopathy*
Examine patient above the umbilicus	*?skin lumps* *?normal respiratory system* *?breast lumps*
Examine the abdomen	*?splenomegaly ?hepatomegaly*

C. Examination of other neck lumps

ACTION	NOTE
Introduce yourself Say what you wish to do Ask the patient's permission to proceed	
Assess as for any lump (pages 41–43)	*?neck triangle* *?shape* *?colour* *?size* *?temperature* *?surface* *?edge* *?consistency*

ACTION	NOTE
Palpate lump as patient contracts the underlying muscle, eg: sternomastoid – tell patient to push chin against your hand (away from the side of the lump); trapezius – tell patient to shrug his or her shoulders as you push down	*?fixation to underlying muscle* *?situated deep to muscle*
Examine for cervical lymphadenopathy (as above)	*?associated lymphadenopathy*

D. Examination of a salivary gland

ACTION	NOTE
Introduce yourself Say what you wish to do Ask the patient's permission to proceed	
Assess as for any lump (pages 41–43)	*?position* *?shape* *?colour* *?size* *?temperature* *?surface* *?edge* *?consistency*

ACTION	NOTE
Look inside the mouth: observe submandibular papillae (on either side of the frenulum) and the parotid duct orifice (opposite the crown of the second upper molar tooth)	duct orifice: ?*inflamed* ?*pus/exudate*
Feel inside the mouth: A box of plastic gloves nearby to bimanually palpate suggests that this is a suspected submandibular gland	?*relation to tongue* ?*relation to floor of mouth* ?*tenderness*
Feel along duct If you suspect enlargement of the parotid gland, test cranial nerve VII: 'screw up your eyes; blow out your cheeks; whistle'	?*stone* ?*facial nerve palsy*

TYPICAL CASES

1. MIDLINE NECK SWELLINGS

You should memorise a list of midline neck swellings as shown below.

Common	• Thyroid swellings
	• Thyroglossal cyst
Uncommon	• Lymph nodes
	• Sublingual dermoid cyst
	• Plunging ranula
	• Pharyngeal pouch
	• Subhyoid bursa
	• Carcinoma of larynx/trachea/oesophagus

Case 1: goitre

Revise the causes of a goitre.

a. Physiological

• Puberty

• Pregnancy.

b. Simple colloid goitre and multinodular goitre

Note: these have the same underlying pathogenesis and a *multifactorial aetiology*:

• Goitrogens

• Dyshormogenesis

• Iodine deficiency (epidemic, endemic)

• Autoimmune.

c. Autoimmune thyroid disease

• Hashimoto's thyroiditis

- Graves' disease.

d. Other thyroiditides

- De Quervain's thyroiditis (acute)
- Riedel's thyroiditis (chronic fibrosing).

e. Tumours

- Benign
- Malignant: primary (carcinoma); secondary (lymphoma).

f. Other

- Tuberculosis
- Sarcoidosis.

Note that if you feel a single nodule you may be feeling the following:

- One nodule of a multinodular goitre
- An enlarged lobe (eg malignant infiltration; Hashimoto's thyroiditis)
- A true single nodule, ie a neoplasm. This may be *benign* (adenoma: functional or non-functional) or *malignant.*

You may be asked about the different kinds of primary thyroid cancers shown below.

Type	Note
Papillary	Anterolateral lump: otherwise known as 'lateral aberrant thyroid'; may actually be an involved lymph node; slow growing
Follicular	Ask about bone pain (metastasises via blood)
Medullary	Lump feels stony-hard due to amyloid infiltration
Anaplastic	Usually middle-aged or elderly patients; not a discrete lump because of infiltration into surrounding tissues, rapid growth, Horner's
Malignant lymphoma	Associated with long-standing Hashimoto's thyroiditis

Assess thyroid status independently: you are expected to know the common causes of hyper- and hypothyroidism.

	Cause	Note
Hyperthyroidism	Graves' disease	• Autoimmune • Younger patients • Goitre is diffusely enlarged with bruit
	Multinodular goitre	• Older patients
	Functioning adenoma	• Rare • Most are non-functioning
Hypothyroidism	Primary myxoedema	• Autoimmune • Older patients • No goitre
	Hashimoto's thyroiditis	• Autoimmune • Younger patients • Rubbery goitre • At an early stage patient may be hyperthyroid

Investigation: determine levels of TSH, T_3 and T_4 (euthyroid: normal TSH; hyperthyroid: TSH $\downarrow T_3 \uparrow$; hypothyroid TSH $\uparrow T_4 \downarrow$), thyroid antibodies for thyroiditis, ultrasonography to differentiate cystic and nodular disease, CT and MRI to identify infiltration, fine-needle aspiration and histological examination.

Treatment:

1. Iodine for deficiency.

2. Remove goitrogens.

3. Suppress TSH with thryoxine in multinodular goitres (can lead to 70% reduction in size).

4. Surgery for retrosternal extension, tracheal compression and malignant tumours.

5.   Anti-thyroid treatment for hyperthyroidism (usually long-term carbimazole with the addition of propranolol in severe cases). Surgery for relapse, if age <40 years; radioiodine in older patients, add 2-week course of Lugol's iodine to drug management preoperatively.

6.   Pregnancy: change antithyroid treatment to thiouracil; surgery safest in second trimester.

Case 2: thyroglossal cyst

This is a spherical midline lump. It feels hard and the edge is clearly defined. It moves with swallowing, but ask the patient to stick out his or her tongue: the lump will move *up* due to its attachment to the fibrous remnants of the thyroglossal tract; this differentiates it from a thyroid mass.

Note its position: is it suprahyoid or infrahyoid?

You may find it difficult to fluctuate and to transilluminate.

Clinical diagnosis aided by imaging, particularly the need to define glossal extension.

Investigation: the clinical diagnosis is aided by imaging, which is particularly important in defining glossal extension.

Treatment: excision of cyst and whole tract. This may loop behind the hyoid bone, requiring resection of the body and following the tract into the base of the tongue.

2. LATERAL NECK SWELLINGS

Don't forget that an asymmetrical thyroid swelling may appear as a lateral neck swelling.

Otherwise, think of a lateral swelling as derived from paired lateral structures. Don't forget that lymph nodes are by far the most common cause.

	Anterior triangle	Posterior triangle
Lymph nodes	• Lymph node • Cold abscess[a]	• Lymph node • Cold abscess[a]
Salivary glands	• Submandibular swelling • Parotid swelling	
Cystic structures	Branchial cyst	Cystic hygroma
Vascular structures	• Carotid body tumour • Carotid artery aneurysm	Subclavian artery aneurysm
Other structures	Sternomastoid 'tumour' (ischaemic contracture)	Tumour of clavicle

[a]Note: a cold abscess arises from TB involvement of the nodes: the caseating nodes *point*, weakening the overlying tissue and then *burst*, causing a 'collar-stud' abscess.

Case 3: cervical lymphadenopathy

You are likely to be asked the differential diagnosis.

	Localised lymphadenopathy	Generalised lymphadenopathy
Infective	• Tonsillitis • Laryngitis • Infected skin lesion, eg sebaceous cyst • TB • Toxoplasmosis	Acute • Infectious mononucleosis • Cytomegalovirus Chronic • TB • Brucellosis • Secondary syphilis • HIV
Neoplastic	Metastases from carcinoma of: • Head and neck • Breast • Chest • Abdomen	Lymphoma • Hodgkin's • Non-Hodgkin's Leukaemias, eg chronic lymphocytic leukaemia
Other		• Amyloidosis • Sarcoidosis

Treatment: identify the aetiology by clinical diagnosis which may be aided by fine-needle aspiration or excision biopsy; search for primary site.

Case 4: salivary gland swelling

You may be given a patient with enlargement of the parotid or submandibular glands. Note how long, changing features, pain.

Be able to classify the causes of salivary gland enlargement:

a. Infection (sialoadenitis)

Acute

- Viral

- Bacterial.

Recurrent

- Obstructive: calculus, stricture

- Non-obstructive: children, menopausal women.

Chronic

- Tuberculosis

- Actinomycosis.

b. Autoimmune

- Sicca syndrome

- Sjögren syndrome.

c. Calculi (sialolithiasis)

d. Cysts

- Simple cysts (parotid)

- Mucus retention cysts.

e. Infiltration

- Sarcoidosis.

f. Systemic disease

- Alcoholic liver cirrhosis

- Diabetes mellitus

- Pancreatitis

- Acromegaly

- Malnutrition.

g. Drugs

- Phenothiazines

- Phenylbutazone.

h. Allergy

- Iodine.

i. Malignancy

- Benign

- Intermediate

- Malignant.

Remember:

- 80% of salivary *neoplastic* conditions occur in the parotid gland.

- Most *stones* occur in the *submandibular* gland.

The most likely cause of parotid enlargement is a benign mixed parotid tumour. Occasionally you will see a Warthin's tumour. The following characteristics distinguish these two tumours.

	Mixed parotid tumour (pleomorphic adenoma)	Warthin's tumour
Position	Just above and anterior to the angle of the jaw	Slightly lower: lower border of mandible
Consistency	Rubbery-hard	Soft
Mobility	+	++
Fluctuant?	No	Yes

You may be asked how you would clinically assess the *malignancy* of a parotid tumour. The distinguishing features are:

- Short presentation

- Painful

- Hyperaemic and hot skin

- Hard consistency

- Fixed to skin and underlying muscle

- Irregular surface and indistinct edge

- Invasion of facial nerve with facial palsy.

Treatment: treat infection with appropriate antibiotic. Dilate strictures, remove stones and marsupialise orifice. Watch small benign tumours. In parotid surgery for benign pleomorphic adenomas, protect facial nerve and aim for conservative resection (eg superficial parotidectomy). Total parotidectomy and facial nerve sacrifice may be performed for infiltrating / malignant lesions. This is associated with neck dissection and lymphadenectomy to remove involved nodes with or without adjunctive radiotherapy.

Case 5: cervical rib

This rarely comes up in examinations.

The lump is only occasionally palpable, just above the clavicle. It may be pulsatile due to the elevated and sometimes dilated subclavian artery.

Look out for neurological and vascular features.

a. Neurological features (more common)

- Pain in C8 and T1 dermatomes

- Wasting and weakness of the small muscles of the hand.

b. Vascular features (rarer)

- Raynaud's phenomenon

- Rest pain

- Trophic changes

- Gangrene.

Treatment: excise symptomatic ribs. Associated vascular lesions may require local resection of aneurysm, distal thrombectomy and sympathectomy.

Case 6: carotid body tumour

This is a rare condition but may come up in the examination as a short case. The tumour feels hard and is sometimes known as a 'potato tumour'. The position is shown in the figure below.

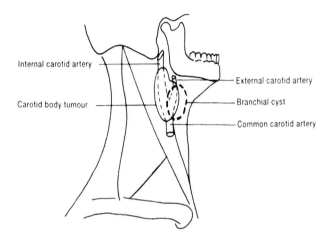

You may feel pulsation. This may result from the following sources:

- Internal carotid artery (transmitted)

- External carotid artery (running superficially)

- Tumour itself (intrinsic vascularity).

Ask about blackouts, transient paralysis and paraesthesia. Check the other side – the tumour is often bilateral.

Treatment: observe small, often bilateral tumours. Excise enlarging, symptomatic and invasive tumours. May need replacement of carotid artery. Essential to make the diagnosis preoperatively so that a vascular surgeon is involved.

Case 7: branchial cyst/sinus/fistula

Note that although these are *developmental*, arising from remnants of the second pharyngeal pouch, they present in young adults.

The cyst has a distinct edge and a smooth surface. Depending on its contents, it may or may not transilluminate.

You may be shown a branchial sinus or fistula – a small dimple in the skin, at the junction of the middle and lower thirds of the anterior edge of sternomastoid:

- Ask the patient to swallow: this will make it more obvious

- Ask about discharge.

Know the *definitions* of a sinus and a fistula:

a. **Sinus:** a blindly-ending track, leading away from an epithelial surface into surrounding tissue, lined by epithelial or granulation tissue. (In this instance there is no closing off of the second branchial cleft, although the upper end is obliterated.)

b. **Fistula:** an abnormal tract connecting two epithelial surfaces, lined by epithelial or granulation tissue. (In this instance the fistula connects skin to the oropharynx, just behind the tonsil.)

Treatment: complete excision.

FAQS AND POPULAR VIVA QUESTIONS

1. What are the causes of cervical lymphadenopathy?

2. What are the possible causes of a lump in the anterior triangle of the neck?

3. What are the causes of a thyroid swelling?

4. What are the causes of hyper- and hypothyroidism?

5. What are the indications for the surgical management of hyperthyroidism?

6. What precautions would you take in preparing a patient with hyperthyroidism for surgery?

7. What are the complications of thyroidectomy?

8. What kinds of thyroid malignancy do you know?

9. What are the sites of the openings of the submandibular and parotid ducts into the mouth?

10. What are the causes of stones in the salivary ducts? Where are they most likely to form?

11. What is the most common tumour of the parotid gland? How should it be managed?

12. What clinical features distinguish a benign from a malignant salivary tumour?

13. What are the complications of surgery to the parotid gland?

ANSWERS

1. (a) Infection: from the skin of the head and neck, the tonsils, adenoids and throat, other sites in the ear and nose, paranasal air sinuses, pharynx and larynx. (b) Part of generalised lymphadenopathy: acute (eg infectious mononucleosis, cytomegalovirus) or chronic (eg TB, brucellosis, secondary syphilis, HIV). (c) Malignancy: primary (eg lymphoma, Hodgkin's lymphoma and leukaemias) or secondary (eg metastases from carcinoma of the head and neck, breast, chest and abdomen). (d) Amyloid and sarcoid infiltration.

2. The **anterior triangle** lies anterior to the sternomastoid muscle below the mandible. The triangles from each side meet in the midline. Lymph nodes and abscesses such as tuberculous ones, salivary glands (submandibular and parotid), carotid body tumours, carotid aneurysms, branchial cysts and tumours of the sternomastoid.

   Midline swellings may appear in either anterior triangle: thyroid swellings, thryoglossal cysts, sublingual dermoid cyst, plunging ranula, pharyngeal pouch, subhyoid bursa and carcinomas of the larynx, trachea and oesophagus.

3. Physiological enlargement at puberty and pregnancy; simple and multiple colloid that may be associated with goitrogens; dyshormogenesis; iodine deficiency; autoimmune thyroid disease (Hashimoto's thyroiditis and Graves' disease); other thyroid disease (de Quervain's and Riedel's thyroiditis); tumours: benign and malignant (primary or secondary); tuberculosis; sarcoidosis.

4. **Hyperthyroidism:** Graves' disease (autoimmune; younger patients with diffusely enlarged goitre and bruit), multinodular goitre (in older patients), toxic adenoma and excessive thyroxine replacement. Rare causes: metastatic thyroid carcinoma, TSH-secreting pituitary tumour, choriocarcinoma, hydatidiform mole and neonatal thyrotoxicosis.
   Hypothyroidism: primary myxoedema (autoimmune; older patients with no goitre), Hashimoto's thyroiditis, over-zealous treatment with drugs, surgery or radioiodine. Neonatal cases: agenesis or maternal anti-thyroid agents.

5. Failure of medical treatment; retrosternal extension and tracheal compression; symptoms of multinodular enlargement. Note that surgical treatment is safest in the middle trimester of pregnancy.

6. Continuation of long-term carbimazole or other anti-thyroid agents; additional propranolol in severe cases and uncontrolled cardiovascular symptoms; Lugol's iodine 2 weeks preoperatively.

7. Immediate complications: acute tracheal obstruction from haematoma, thyroid crisis, recurrent laryngeal nerve damage. Longer-term complications: hypocalcaemia from parathyroid excision, long-term hypothyroidism and recurrent hyperthyroidism.

8. Papillary and follicular carcinoma, medullary carcinoma (associated with multiple endocrine neoplasia types IIa and IIb), anaplastic carcinoma and aggressive neoplasms (of middle-aged and elderly patients) and malignant lymphomas (associated with long-standing Hashimoto's thyroiditis).

9. **Submandibular:** in the floor of the mouth on the submandibular papilla, situated on each side of the frenulum of the tongue. The **parotid** duct opens opposite the crown of the second upper molar tooth.

10. Stenosis in the duct due to chronic infection and oral disease around the papilla. They usually occur in the **submandibular gland**, leading to pain and distension on eating; very rarely found in the parotid gland.

11. **Pleomorphic adenoma** – commonest parotid tumour: small non-progressive tumours – regular observation. Superficial parotidectomy or excision with a surrounding cuff of normal tissue is the surgical alternative. The more extensive excision requires particular care of the facial nerve. Occasionally radiotherapy is required for recurrent problems.

12. **Benign:** smooth, lobulated, painless, may be bilateral, when superficial may be slightly mobile, usually soft to firm, slowly enlarging over years. **Malignant:** firm to hard, fixed, rapid growth over a number of months, facial nerve involvement and infiltration of surrounding tissues.

13. **Facial nerve injury** (which may be unavoidable in treating malignant disease), Frey syndrome, gustatory sweating due to divided parasymphathetic nerves growing into the skin, salivary fistula, recurrence of malignancy.

9 | The breast

Your patient in either the long or short case might be a woman complaining of pain (cyclical, persistent, progressive) or a lump in her breast.

THE HISTORY

Bring out the following points when presenting under 'history of presenting complaint'.

Breast lump

- When did you notice the lump? How did you notice it?

- Has the lump *changed* since you first noticed it? How?

- Is it painful?

- Have you had any breast lumps in the past?

- Has anyone in your family had breast lumps?

Hormonal factors

- Does the lump change with your menstrual cycle or at different times in the month?

- When did you start your periods? (*menarche*) If relevant – When did you stop your periods? (*menopause*)

- How many children do you have? Did you breast-feed them? Were there any problems?

- Have you ever been on the pill or hormone replacement therapy?

Nipple discharge

- Spontaneous or elicited?
- Do you have discharge from *both* nipples?
- What colour is the discharge?
- Have you breast-fed recently?

THE EXAMINATION

The usual instruction given in the short case is to 'examine the breasts'. Proceed as below (a chaperone should be present, and may be requested).

Occasionally, you may be asked just to feel and describe a lump in the breast, in which case you should proceed as described on pages 41–43. Remember at all times to be sensitive and to avoid embarrassment and discomfort. Cover the breasts up when you are examining other systems.

'Examine this patient's breasts'

ACTION	NOTE
Introduce yourself	
Say what you wish to do	
Ask the patient's permission to proceed	
Expose the breasts; first examine with patient sitting on side of couch	
LOOK	
Stand opposite the patient	
First observe with arms at side	
Ask her to raise her arms slowly above her head	*?asymmetry*
	?skin puckering
Ask her to lean forward	*?dimpling, other change*
In this postion ask her to lean forward and then to press her hands on hips	*?nipple deviation retraction, eczema*
	axillary lumps

ACTION	NOTE
FEEL	If your patient has pendulous breasts, lie her flatter. Rest the arm of the breast to be examined behind her head. Ask her to lean slightly to the other side, supported by a pillow
Ask the patient to point to the lump with one finger	
Ask if the breasts are tender	
Start with the normal breast	
Palpate *systematically*, each quadrant in turn, and then centrally around the nipple	
Palpate with the flat of your fingers	
Palpate the *affected* breast: all quadrants except that of the lump itself	
ASSESS THE LUMP	Omit this section if no lump is found on examination
Feel and measure the lump	overlying skin: ?*warm, red*
	texture: ?*stony-hard*
	?*rubbery-hard*
	?*soft*
	shape/size: ?*exact dimensions*
Try to move the skin overlying the lump	skin: ?*no movement* (implies fixation)
	?*wrinkles at extremes of movement* (implies tethering)
	peau d'orange, ulceration

ACTION	NOTE
Ask your patient to rest her hand lightly on the hip of the same side. Move the lump with your finger and thumb:	
• up and down	*?mobility*
• at right angles	
Ask her to press hard on her hip	
Move the lump as above	movement of lump: *?reduces on contraction of pectoral muscles* (indicates attachment to muscle)
Try to elicit any discharge by gently squeezing the nipple (warn patient)	site: *?nipple segment*
	colour: *?red*
	?green
	?yellow
	?clear
REPEAT THE EXAMINATION OF THE OTHER BREAST	
Examine the axillae: hold the patient's right elbow in your right hand	
Take the weight of her forearm	
Palpate the walls with your left hand:	If in doubt, palpate posteriorly and laterally from behind patient
• medial	
• anterior	
• lateral	*?associated lymphadenopathy*
• posterior	
• apical	
Repeat on the other side, changing hands	

ACTION	NOTE
Palpate the cervical nodes	
Palpate the supraclavicular fossae and behind sternomastoid	
ASSESS FURTHER	
Palpate the liver	*?hepatomegaly*
	?knobbly edge
Percuss down the back	*?tenderness,* suggestive of bone metastases
Ask if it is tender at any point	
Percuss the lung bases	*?dull,* suggestive of consolidation or effusion
COMPLETE THE EXAMINATION	
Cover the patient's breasts with a sheet	
Turn to the examiner and present your findings	

TYPICAL CASES

Breast lumps come up as long (OSLER) and short (OSCE) cases. Revise the causes of a breast lump.

Cause	Example	
Physiological	Fibroadenosis	
Neoplastic	*Benign*	• Fibroadenoma
		• Duct papilloma
		• Phylloides tumour
	Malignant	• Primary carcinoma
		• Secondary carcinoma
Traumatic	Fat necrosis	
Infective	Cellulitis	
	Abscesses	

You should be able to differentiate clinically between the more common lumps.

	Carcinoma	Fibroadenoma	Fibroadenosis
No. of lumps	1	1+	1+
Pain	Rare	Rare	Common: varies with menstrual cycle
Irregularity	++	–	–
Hardness	+++	++	+

Case 1: breast carcinoma

This is a very common case. Remember the classic features.

a. Age 35+

b. Positive family history

c. Lump

- Stony-hard
- Irregular edge
- Tethered vs fixed to skin? (see table opposite)
- Immobile
- Peau d'orange.

d. Nipple

- Inverted
- Distorted
- Bloody discharge
- Red, encrusted, oozing (Paget's disease).

e. Lymphadenopathy

f. Features of metastases

- Backache
- Breathlessness
- Jaundice
- Malaise and weight loss.

	Tethering	Fixation
Infiltration	Along ligaments of Astley Cooper	To skin
Mobility	Some	None
Skin	Dimples at extremes of movement	Cannot be moved over lump
Prognosis	Better	Worse

Remember that the signs of breast carcinoma may be mimicked by other conditions. Consider the following:

a. Hard irregular lumps: fat necrosis and chronic mastitis.

b. Nipple inversion: this may be long-standing or congenital.

c. Nipple discharge: see Case 4.

d. Nipple skin changes: differentiate Paget's disease from eczema.

	Paget's disease	Eczema
Cause	Spread of intraductal carcinoma to epidermis	Atopy
Bilateral?	No	Yes
Itchy?	No	Yes
Vesicular?	No	Yes

Screening: in the UK all women aged 50–70 are invited for breast cancer screening every 3 years. This involves a bilateral breast X-ray (mammogram). This aims to detect breast cancers early and offer curative surgical treatment.

Staging: staging of breast cancer is valuable both in choice of treatment and as a prognostic indicator. Stages 1–4 have a TNM classification superimposed.

Stage 1: early disease confined to the breast (T1 <2 cm) or Paget's disease

Stage 2: axillary nodal spread (T2 2–5 cm, N1); stages 1 and 2 are classified as early disease

Stage 3a: locally advanced disease

Stage 3b: chest wall involvement (T3 >5 cm, T4 skin and chest wall involvement, N2 fixed nodes, N3 ipsilateral internal mammary nodes)

Stage 4: extension of disease beyond the breast (M1).

Treatment: (extensive National and International guidelines exist for management of breast cancer; know your hospital's current policy)

1. Early lesions require complete surgical excision with negative margins. According to lesion size, this surgical excision can involve a lumpectomy, segmental mastectomy or modified radical mastectomy. More recent techniques include skin-sparing or nipple-sparing mastectomy in selected patients.

2. Breast reconstruction can occur at the time of primary surgery or as a separate procedure. Different techniques include transverse rectus abdominus myocutaneous flap (TRAM) or a deep inferior epigastric perforator flap (DIEP).

3. Local radiotherapy is administered to reduce the risk of local recurrence.

4. Assessment of axillary lymph node involvement is essential. This is performed by injection of radioisotopes in the breast and selective excision of axillary lymph nodes showing high isotope uptake (hence predominant tumour drainage). This technique is known as sentinel lymph node biopsy. It aims to prevent the co-morbidities associated with axillary clearance (eg arm lymphoedema) or unreliability of axillary sampling.

5. Adjuvant therapy for breast cancers includes:

   a. Chemotherapy

   b. Hormonal therapy for patients that are oestrogen-receptor positive: selective oestrogen-receptor modulator (tamoxifen) or aromatase inhibitors

   c. Immunotherapy for patients over-expressing *HER2* using monoclonal antibodies (trastuzumab)

6. Advanced lesions require mastectomy with axillary lymph node clearance together with a patient-specific combination of adjuvant therapy. Palliation is given to patients where curative therapy is not possible.

The Nottingham Prognostic Index (NPI) uses: the size of the lesion; tumour grade; number of involved lymph nodes. A score of ≤ 3.4 with the system suggests an 85% 5-year survival and > 5.4 a 50% survival rate.

Case 2: fibroadenoma

A woman with a fibroadenoma will usually be young (peak 25–35 years).

There may be more than one lump. The lumps are small and rubbery-hard. They are very mobile and are therefore also known as 'breast mice'.

Investigation: includes ultrasonography and fine-needle cytology (these with the clinical examination comprise the 'triple assessment').

Treatment: refer to specialist breast unit for triple assessment. Excision biopsy may be subsequently recommended to exclude malignancy, although simple, low-risk lesions that have been triply assessed can be monitored radiologically.

Case 3: fibroadenosis

Terminology varies: aberration of normal development and involution (ANDI) most accurately describes the process.

This condition is very common and borders on physiological change.

It occurs in women of reproductive age, peak 35–45 years. Ask specifically about variation with the menstrual cycle.

There are many presentations:

- Single lump (solid or cystic)
- Multiple lumps or generalised nodularity
- Cyclical breast pain
- Nipple discharge (clear, white or green).

Investigation and treatment: age <35–40; ultrasound; age >40, mammography to exclude neoplasia. Stop hormonal contraceptives or HRT. A trial of evening primrose oil. Where cysts have been aspirated, core needle biopsy or excision biopsy is used to assess any residual lesion.

Case 4: nipple discharge

Ask yourself the following key questions:

a. Is the discharge a true discharge?

Eczema, Paget's disease and fistulae all cause discharges that do not arise from the ducts themselves.

b. Is the discharge significant?

For a discharge to be significant, it must have occurred:

- Spontaneously

- Over a year after stopping breast-feeding

- More than once.

c. Is the discharge worrying?

The following features suggest carcinoma:

- *Unilateral* discharge

- *Bloody* discharge

- Discharge arising from a *single* duct (single nipple segment).

The colour of the discharge may give you a clue as to the cause.

Colour	Nature	Cause
Red	Blood	• Ductal carcinoma • Duct papilloma
Green	Cell debris	• Fibroadenosis • Duct ectasia
Yellow	Exudate	• Fibroadenosis • Abscess
White	Milk	• Lactation

Investigation: includes cytology of the discharge and triple assessment (palpation, breast imaging and fine-needle cytology of any underlying lesion). This is followed by core needle biopsy of any area of equivocal findings.

Treatment: malignancy is managed as outlined in Case 1 or enrolment onto a screening programme, based on these investigation results.

FAQS AND POPULAR VIVA QUESTIONS

1. What is a fibroadenoma?

2. How can fibroadenosis present?

3. What benign breast diseases come into the differential diagnosis of breast cancer?

4. What are the advantages of mammography for breast cancer screening?

5. What are the presenting features of breast carcinoma?

6. Where does breast cancer spread to?

7. What is Paget's disease of the nipple?

8. What are the causes of nipple discharge?

9. What do you understand by the term 'early breast cancer'?

10. How would you manage a woman with early breast cancer?

11. What are the advantages of lumpectomy over mastectomy for breast cancer?

12. What is advanced breast cancer?

13. What are the alternative treatments in advanced breast cancer?

ANSWERS

1. A focal area of lobular stromal hyperplasia with epithelial proliferation.

2. Non-cyclical breast discomfort with or without swelling or nodularity. When present, nodularity may be both palpable and tender, and may include cystic changes.

3. Fibroadenoma, fibroadenosis, acute and chronic infection, fat necrosis, sclerosing adenonis, granulomatous lobular and periductal mastitis, and eczematous disease of the nipple.

4. Mammography screening of the female population at age 50–70 may detect non-palpable asymptomatic disease. Serial assessment at 3-year intervals may identify early malignant change. Abnormalities are detected by specialist teams. Triple assessment (clinical, imaging, tissue sampling) is recommended.

5. Of symptomatic lesions, 80% present with a palpable lump, nipple retraction or a blood-strained discharge; axillary mass or Paget's disease is less common; asymptomatic disease may be picked up on screening.

6. Local spread may distort the nipple, tethering to skin may produce peau d'orange and deep tethering may cause fixation. Nodal spread is to the axilla and is frequently to the internal mammary nodes. Vascular spread is primarily to the liver, lung and bone.

7. Paget's disease of the nipple is a subepidermoid carcinoma arising in the nipple/areola complex, presenting with eczema of the nipple.

8. Bloody discharge from a ductal papilloma and carcinoma; green cell debris from fibroadenosis and duct ectasia; yellow exudate from fibroadenosis and abscesses; milk from the lactating breast. Cutaneous discharge may arise from eczematous change.

9/10.

   Early breast disease is stage 1 (TI: a tumour of <2 cm) and stage 2 (T2: 2–5 cm); if axillary nodes are present, they must be mobile. Treatment involves complete local excision of lesions of <5 cm as well as radiotherapy to the conserved breast; after initial sentinel node biopsy and frozen section, a decision is made on axillary surgery; axillary clearance below the axillary vein and medial to the pectoralis minor muscle.

11. Lumpectomy conserves breast tissue but requires prophylactic radiotherapy.

12/13.

Advanced cancer is stage 3 (tumours of >5cm: T3), or extension into the skin or chest wall (T4). Axillary nodes are fixed (N2), ipsilateral internal mammary nodes are present (N3) and stage 4 extension beyond the breast and chest wall (M1). Treatment is based on national guidelines and involves a multidisciplinary team, it may include radiotherapy, endocrine therapy and chemotherapy directed at symptomatic, local and distal sites.

10 The gastrointestinal tract

THE HISTORY

Give a succinct and chronological report of your patient's presenting complaint. Bring out the following aspects in your presentation.

The history of the patient's pain

See page 25.

The history of the patient's lump/swelling

See page 40.

Remainder of systemic enquiry of the GIT

Ask about the following symptoms:

- Dysphagia/dyspepsia
- Abdominal swelling/distension/pain
- Nausea and vomiting/flatulence, haematemesis
- Appetite and weight loss
- Change in bowel habit, rectal bleeding
- Jaundice, pruritis
- Overseas travel
- Family history of bowel problems.

Remember that diarrhoea/constipation are not precise words: ask what is normal for your patient.

Report on the stool:

- *?consistency*

- *?frequency, quantity*

- *?colour*

- *?offensive*

- *?blood (?mixed in, on the surface, on the toilet paper)*

- *?mucus/slime*

- *?anal discharge/pruritus ani/tenderness.*

THE EXAMINATION

Listen carefully to the instruction. In a short case, you may be asked to 'examine the gastrointestinal system' or 'examine the abdomen'.

As with the examination of any system, always start with the hands. You may be stopped at this stage and asked to proceed to the abdomen itself. Occasionally, you may be instructed to 'palpate the abdomen', in which case beginning with the hands will only antagonise the examiners.

Note the following points:

- Make sure that your hands are warm.

- Don't hurt your patient: ask if an area is tender during palpation; keep looking at his or her face for wincing.

- Don't forget the following points on account of exam nerves:

    - percussion of the upper border of the liver (*normally fifth intercostal space; may be displaced downwards with hyperexpansion of the chest*)

    - groin

    - external genitalia

    - statement that you would normally perform a rectal examination.

Also remember the **3 A**s:

1. **A**ortic aneurysm

2. **A**scites

3. **A**uscultation.

'Examine this patient's gastrointestinal system'

ACTION	NOTE
Introduce yourself	
Say what you wish to do	
Ask the patient's permission to proceed	
Expose the abdomen with the patient lying flat with one pillow supporting the patient's head	Include the inguinal regions but not the genitalia

1. Preliminary assessment

ACTION	NOTE	
Look at both hands	nails:	*?clubbing*
		?leukonychia
		?koilonychia
		?splinter haemorrhages
	palms:	*?palmar erythema*
		?Dupuytren's contracture
		?pallor of skin creases
	dorsum:	*?tattoos*

ACTION	NOTE
	?bruising, purpura
	?spider naevi
Ask patient to stretch out arms with the wrists cocked up	*?liver flap*
Look at the eyes	sclera: *?jaundice*
	conjunctiva: *?pallor*
Look at the mouth	*?telangiectasia* (indicates hereditary haemorrhagic telangiectasia)
	?perioral pigmentation (indicates Peutz–Jeghers syndrome)
	?ulceration
	?gingivitis
	?caries
Look at the angles of the mouth	*?angular stomatitis* (can occur in young people, but sign of iron deficiency and debilitation in old people)
Ask patient to stick out tongue	*?dehydration*
	?coated tongue
Smell breath	*?ketosis*
	?halitosis
	?uraemic hepatic failure
Palpate supraclavicular lymph nodes	In this case, it is not necessary to examine from behind the patient
	?cervical lymphadenopathy
Show the examiner that you are paying particular attention to the *left* supraclavicular fossa	*?Virchow's node/Troisier's sign*
Look at the chest	skin: *?spider naevi*

ACTION	NOTE
	?purpura
	?gynaecomastia

2. The abdomen

ACTION	NOTE	
LOOK/INSPECT		
Stand at the end of the bed	skin:	*?scars*
		?stoma site
		?visible veins
	shape:	*?distended*
		?scaphoid
		?visible peristalsis
		?visible organs
		?visible masses/hernias
Ask patient to take a deep breath, draw in the abdomen and cough, to blow out the abdomen	*?pain* (limiting movement) *?asymmetry* (mass, discomfort) *?mass* (made more obvious)	
Ask the patient to lean forward	*?nephrectomy/thoracotomy scars*	
FEEL/PALPATE		
Palpate with your palm and the flat of your fingers	You may need to kneel down if the bed is low	
Keep your forearm level with the abdominal wall		

ACTION	NOTE
a. Preliminary palpation	
Ask if the abdomen is tender	
Palpate each quadrant lightly	*?tenderness*
	?guarding
	?rigidity
Palpate each quadrant more deeply, leaving the tender areas until last	*?deep tenderness*
	?masses
	?palpable viscera
b. Assessment of a mass	
If you find a mass, determine its characteristics at this stage (pages 41–43)	*?size*
	?shape
	?surface
	?edge
	?consistency
	?percussion note
	?bruit/bowel sounds
c. Assessment of organomegaly	
Liver	
Palpate the liver, beginning in the right iliac fossa	*?hepatomegaly*
As patient breathes in and out, move your hand upwards in stages until you reach the costal margin	*?smooth edge*
	?knobbly edge
	?consistency
	?tenderness
	?pulsatility
Percuss out the liver: lower and upper borders	*?dull*

ACTION	NOTE
Spleen	
Palpate the spleen, beginning in the right iliac fossa	?*splenomegaly*
As patient breathes in and out, move your hand towards the tip of the tenth rib	
On reaching the costal margin, place your left hand around the lower left rib cage	If you still cannot feel the spleen, ask the patient to roll towards you
Palpate with your right hand in the midaxillary line	
Percuss for an enlarged spleen	?*dull*
Kidneys	
Palpate each kidney: position one hand behind patient's loin and the other hand just above ASIS	Your hand should be *well* behind patient's loin
Ask patient to breath deeply	?*enlarged kidneys*
Aortic aneurysm	
Place two hands on either side of the midline, just above the umbilicus	?*expansile pulsation* ?*can you get above it* (if so, probably infrarenal) ?*transverse diameter*
d. Examination of groin and external genitalia	(see pages 125, 139)
Place your fingers over the inguinal and femoral orifices	?*cough impulse*
Ask patient to cough	
Feel inguinal lymph nodes	?*inguinal lymphadenopathy*
Feel testes	?*atrophy* ?*mass*

ACTION	NOTE
e. Examination for ascites	This is necessary only if the abdomen is distended
Shifting dullness	
Percuss over the abdomen	Keep your finger in the sagittal plane
Start centrally and move to the flanks	
Locate the point on one side where the percussion note changes from resonant to dull	
Ask patient to roll over on that side, keeping your hand in this position	
Percuss again	*?has area of dullness moved (shifting dullness)*
Ask patient to place the edge of his or her hand along the midline	
Flick one side while feeling the other	*?fluid thrill*
LISTEN	
Auscultate abdomen over at least three different areas	*?bowel sounds* (absent, tinkling) *?pitch* *?increased/decreased*
Listen along the course of the aorta and iliac arteries and in the renal areas	*?bruits*
Over liver	*haemangioma; venous hum of portosystemic shunt*

ACTION	NOTE
SAY	
'I would like to:	
• examine the external genitalia	(see page 139)
• do a rectal examination	*?mass*
• examine the urine with a dipstick'	*?proteinuria*
	?haematuria
	?glucose
COMPLETE THE EXAMINATION	
Cover the patient up	
Turn to the examiner	
Present your findings	

TYPICAL CASES

You are unlikely to meet a patient with an acute abdomen in either the short or the long case. However, you should revise the causes of acute abdominal pain for discussion in the clinical examination and viva.

In the long case, you may meet patients with abdominal symptoms but few signs. Examples are patients with peptic ulcers, chronic cholecystitis (and bouts of biliary colic), chronic pancreatitis, diverticular disease, irritable bowel syndrome and inflammatory bowel disease.

You may also have a patient with jaundice. In a surgical examination, the most likely cause will be post-hepatic 'obstructive' jaundice. However, when asked the differential diagnosis, mention pre-hepatic and hepatocellular causes.

The main physical signs, to be picked up in both the long and the short case, are scars and stomas, organomegaly, masses and distension. This section revises the differential diagnosis of these signs.

1. SCARS AND STOMAS

Scars

Always look very carefully for abdominal scars: old ones are surprisingly easy to miss, especially in hirsute men. It is particularly easy to miss a Pfannenstiel incision, appendicectomy scar and a left nephrectomy scar (look well over the left loin).

You should know the usual sites shown in the figure.

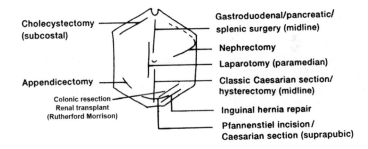

Short (1–1.5-cm) scars in the umbilical region, along the midline and elsewhere may indicate laparoscopic procedures.

Stomas

You should understand the differences between ileostomies and colostomies.

	Ileostomy	Colostomy	Urostomy
Shape	Spout	Flush	Spout
Position	Right side	Left side	Either side
Effluent	Brown/green liquid	Brown formed / solid stool	Yellow urine
Types	End ileostomy (post-colectomy) Loop ileostomy (post primary large bowel anastomosis)	End colostomy (post rectal excision)	Following radical cystectomy or pelvic excenteration

2. ORGANOMEGALY

Case 1: hepatomegaly

In a surgical examination, the most common cause of hepatomegaly is metastases. The patient may or may not be jaundiced. Your examiner will expect you to know the other causes of hepatomegaly.

Common causes in the UK include the following:

- Metastases

- Congestive cardiac failure (right-sided)

- Cirrhosis (not in later stages, when liver shrinks and is impalpable)

- Infections, eg viral hepatitis, infectious mononucleosis.

Go through your surgical sieve (page 17) to retrieve rarer causes.

Your *description* of the liver should help in your differential diagnosis:

a. Edge:	(1) *Smooth*	• Cirrhosis • Congestive heart failure
	(2) *Knobbly*	• Secondary carcinoma • Macronodular cirrhosis (rare)

b. Consistency: *hard* if metastases.

c. Tenderness occurs when capsule is distended:

- Congestive heart failure

- Hepatitis

- Hepatocellular carcinoma

- AV malformation

- Alcoholic hepatitis (rare).

d. Pulsatility: tricuspid regurgitation.

See Treatment after Case 3.

Case 2: Splenomegaly

If your patient has splenomegaly, you may well be asked to justify your diagnosis in terms of its five distinguishing characteristics:

1. Descends towards the right iliac fossa

2. Moves down on inspiration

3. Palpable anterior notch

4. Cannot get above it

5. Dull to percussion (continuous with area of splenic dullness over ribs 9, 10 and 11, behind posterior axillary line).

Have a list of causes of massive, moderate and mild splenomegaly. As always, give the common causes in the UK first (eg myelofibrosis rather than kala-azar for massive splenomegaly).

Massive	Moderate	Mild
	As for massive *plus*	As for moderate *plus*
• Myelofibrosis • Chronic granulocytic leukaemia • Malaria • Kala-azar	• Haemolytic anaemia • Chronic lymphocytic leukaemia • Lymphomas • Portal hypertension	• Infectious mononucleosis • Myeloproliferative disorders • Pernicious anaemia • Amyloidosis • Sarcoidosis • Rheumatoid arthritis (Felty syndrome)

Although many of these causes of splenomegaly are 'medical', your patient may be awaiting a splenectomy because of its complications: *hypersplenism* leads to both pooling and destruction of haematopoietic cells by the reticuloendothelial system, causing a pancytopenia. Be aware of the potential problems of splenectomy, eg infection with capsulated bacteria such as pneumococci. Know about the measures to reduce such complications (Pneumovax immunisation, prophylactic penicillin). See Treatment following Case 3.

Case 3: hepatosplenomegaly

Causes of enlargement of the spleen as well as the liver include some of the above, eg lymphoma, leukaemias, infections, amyloidosis and sarcoidosis. The most likely case in an examination is cirrhosis with associated portal hypertension.

Treatment for Cases 1, 2 and 3: management of most of the listed diseases is that of the underlying cause. Surgery for hepatomegaly might include drainage of abscesses, segmental resection of tumours and occasionally transplantation. **Indications for splenectomy** include septicaemic abscesses, schistosomiasis, tropical splenomegaly, hydatid cysts, Gaucher's disease, myelofibrosis, thalassaemia, sickle cell disease, lymphoma, embolic infarction, splenic artery or venous thrombosis, and possibly hereditary spherocytosis, idiopathic splenomegaly, thrombocytopenic purpura and solitary or polycystic disease.

Case 4: enlarged kidneys

Remember that in slim people the lower pole of a normal right kidney may be palpable.

Know the characteristics of a renal swelling:

- Ballotable (*bimanually palpable*)

- Descends vertically

- Moves down on inspiration and can be 'trapped' between your hands

- Resonant to percussion due to overlying colon (*not always*: some parts may be dull)

- Can get above it (*rarely*).

Another popular question is to differentiate between an enlarged left kidney and a palpable spleen,

	Kidney	Spleen
Descent on inspiration?	Vertically	Towards right iliac fossa
Ballotable?	Yes	No
Notch present?	No	Yes
Can you ever get above it?	Occasionally	No
Percussion note?	Resonant (usually)	Dull

In finals, the most common cause of *bilateral* renal enlargement is polycystic kidneys. These may be extremely large and feel lobulated because of the multiple cysts. If you suspect this condition:

• Ask about family history (inheritance is *autosomal dominant*)

• Take the blood pressure

• Ask to examine the urine (?*haematuria*, ?*proteinuria*, ?*casts*) – try to palpate the liver, which might also be polycystic

• Look for a third cranial nerve palsy due to pressure from an associated posterior communicating artery berry aneurysm.

Other causes of bilateral renal enlargement are bilateral hydronephrosis and amyloidosis.

Causes of *unilateral* renal enlargement include the following:

• Hydronephrosis

• Simple benign cysts

• Hypertrophy

• Tumour, eg renal cell carcinoma.

A transplanted kidney is usually found in an iliac fossa.

Treatment: progressive renal failure from polycystic disease may require transplantation; hydronephrosis: drainage and treatment of the cause; renal cell carcinoma: nephrectomy with removal of intravenous extension and possibly pulmonary metastases.

3. MASSES

Revise pages 41–43 for the description of any mass.

As many masses are visible on careful observation of the abdomen, do not forget to look first.

List and revise the causes of masses in each segment of the abdomen.

Case 5: mass in the right hypochondrium

The causes of a mass in the right hypochondrium include the following:

- Hepatomegaly

- Enlarged gallbladder

- Enlarged right kidney

- Colonic mass.

Revise the causes of an enlarged gallbladder:

a. Obstruction of cystic duct: mucocele or empyema.

b. Obstruction of the common bile duct, eg cancer of the head of the pancreas.

Remember *Courvoisier's law*:

'If the gallbladder is palpable and the patient is jaundiced, the obstruction of the bile duct causing the jaundice is unlikely to be due to a stone.' The gallbladder is fibrotic and contracted in inflammatory (non-malignant) disease.

c. Gallbladder mass: inflammation with surrounding adherent omentum

Also note the characteristics of an enlarged gallbladder:

- Appears from the tip of rib 9 and cannot get between it and the liver edge

- Dull to percussion

- Smooth surface

- Moves down on inspiration (not always true of gallbladder mass).

See Treatment following Case 10.

Case 6: mass in the epigastrium

The two most important causes are carcinoma of the stomach and pancreatic masses (pseudocyst, carcinoma). An aortic aneurysm is situated deep to the umbilicus, but may also fill the epigastrium.

Three 'catches' are:

1. **Liver:** either left lobe or a post-necrotic nodule of a cirrhotic liver.

2. **Large recti:** these appear to enlarge when the patient sits forwards.

3. **Prominent xiphisternum:** comes to light at odd ages.

You should suspect gastric or pancreatic carcinoma in a cachectic patient complaining of pain, dyspepsia, anorexia and significant weight loss. You may not always feel a mass.

Note the characteristics of a *gastric* carcinoma:

- Hard, irregular

- Cannot get above it

- Moves with respiration.

Think immediately of checking for a left supraclavicular node (*Virchow's node/Troisier's sign*).

Gastric carcinoma may be difficult to differentiate from a pancreatic pseudocyst which, although uncommon, crops up disproportionately often in examinations. The characteristics of a pancreatic pseudocyst are as follows:

- Cannot get above it

- Indistinct lower border

- Resonant to percussion

- Moves slightly with respiration.

See Treatment following Case 10.

Case 7: mass in the left hypochondrium

The most common cause is an enlarged spleen. Other causes are a pancreatic mass (carcinoma of tail) and an enlarged left kidney.

See Treatment following Case 10.

Case 8: mass in the right loin

- Enlarged right kidney

- Enlarged liver

- Enlarged gallbladder.

See Treatment following Case 10.

Case 9: mass in the umbilical region

- Small-bowel mass (nodal or omental)

- Cancer of transverse colon

- Aortic aneurysm.

See Treatment following Case 10.

Case 10: mass in the left loin

- Enlarged left kidney

- Enlarged spleen.

Investigations for Cases 5–10: confirmation of the diagnosis in these areas can usually be obtained by imaging techniques. CT and MRI provide reliable diagnostic information on the liver, spleen, pancreas, kidneys and retroperitoneal structures, identifying inflammatory change as well as benign and malignant tumours, with or without invasion and secondary spread.

Treatment for Cases 5–10:

Aortic aneurysm: an abdominal aortic aneurysm is usually a clinical diagnosis; intervention by stenting or open surgery is considered in lesions >5.5 cm in diameter, or rapidly expanding (all require regular follow-up).

Gallbladder: cholelithiasis is managed by cholecystectomy and exploration and evacuation of the common bile and hepatic ducts, possibly endoscopically.

Pancreas: acute pancreatitis occasionally requires surgical débridement and drainage; malignant tumours of the body and tail of the pancreas are usually inoperable by the time of diagnosis; a lesion causing jaundice might still be resectable using Whipple's procedure.

Case 11: mass in the right iliac fossa

A mass in the right iliac fossa is a common clinical case.

The most common causes are carcinoma of the caecum and Crohn's disease.

a. Carcinoma of caecum

Suspect this condition in an elderly patient who appears clinically anaemic. The mass is often well defined and hard. It can be mobile or fixed. It is not usually tender.

b. Crohn's disease

This is usually seen in younger patients. The mass feels rubbery and non-tender and can be fairly mobile. See Treatment following Case 12.

These are the less common causes:

- Appendix mass

- Ileocaecal TB

- Congenital abnormal kidney

- Infected caecal diverticulum

- Iliac lymphadenopathy

- Ovarian cyst

- Ectopic pregnancy

- Transplanted kidney

- Iliac artery aneurysm.

Case 12: mass in the left iliac fossa

The common causes are a loaded sigmoid colon (can be palpable normally, but, particularly with constipation or diverticular disease, it can be indented) and carcinoma of the colon. Rarer causes are Crohn's disease and iliac lymphadenopathy. Again, don't forget gynaecological causes (eg an ovarian mass) or transplanted kidney.

a. Diverticular disease

You are unlikely to be given a patient with a diverticular abscess. However, patients with diverticular disease often have a palpable, tender sigmoid colon.

b. Carcinoma of colon

The patient normally presents with a change in bowel habit. The mass is usually hard.

Feel for an enlarged liver and listen for high-pitched bowel sounds (in the presence of any obstruction); palpate for enlarged inguinal nodes.

Treatment for Cases 11 and 12: most iliac fossa masses are related to lesions of the colon. Appendix abscesses may require drainage. Those extending laterally are allowed to resolve, followed, after a few months, by interval appendicectomy. Medial extensions may give rise to further gut symptoms and may require a difficult surgical resection in the acute phase.

Obstruction from inflammatory bowel disease, diverticular disease or colonic malignancy may require emergency surgery with temporary colostomy, requiring subsequent resection with or without restoration of gut continuity. It may also be possible to undertake definitive surgery at the time of the initial emergency procedure. Fulminating toxic megacolon in ulcerative colitis is a serious emergency that may respond to steroids. Emergency surgery is directed at retroperitoneal decompression to avoid peritoneal contamination before total proctocolectomy.

Crohn's disease may require drainage of abscesses and resection of fistulae. The aim is to preserve as much bowel as possible.

Case 13: abdominal distension

Remember the **5 F**s:

1. **F**etus: very unlikely in a surgical examination but always consider in a woman of reproductive age.

2. **F**latus: the abdomen is hyper-resonant; you may see visible peristalsis, implying bowel obstruction.

3. **F**aeces: you are unlikely to be given a patient with acute obstruction. However, chronic constipation is a common surgical problem. Beware – your patient may be complaining of diarrhoea and in fact be constipated (spurious diarrhoea). Faeces have the following characteristics:

    – lie in the distribution of the colon

    – often form multiple separate masses

    – can be indented with digital pressure.

4. **F**at: usually obvious; deposition is in the lower half of the abdomen.

5. **F**luid: ascites can be detected by two tests: fluid thrill and shifting dullness. The latter is more reliable because a fluid thrill is detected in any abdominal fluid-filled cavity.

Treatment: according to diagnosis (see treatment of Cases 11 and 12). Initial imaging includes an erect chest X-ray (to rule out bowel perforation) and a plain abdominal X-ray (to rule out bowel distension). Subsequently abdominal CT or ultrasound scanning is usually required. Ascites requires diagnostic aspiration if the cause is unknown. Ascitic fluid needs to be sent for biochemical (exudate / transudate), cytological (benign / malignant) and microbiological (infection) analysis.

FAQS AND POPULAR VIVA QUESTIONS

1. What are the causes of:
   - dysphagia
   - hepatomegaly
   - splenomegaly
   - hepatosplenomegaly
   - jaundice
   - change in bowel habit
   - diarrhoea
   - constipation
   - haematemesis
   - melaena
   - bleeding per rectum
   - intestinal obstruction: *?in children, ?in adults*
   - pruritis ani?

2. Differentiate tenderness, rebound tenderness, guarding and rigidity.

3. What is the difference between peritonism and peritonitis?

4. How do gallstones present?

5. How does presentation of carcinoma of the head of the pancreas differ from that of the tail of the pancreas?

6. What is the difference between diverticulosis and diverticulitis?

7. What are the complications of diverticular disease?

8. What are the differences between Crohn's disease and ulcerative colitis?

9. What are the local and general complications of inflammatory bowel disease?

10. What is Dukes' staging for colorectal cancer?

11. How does the presentation of carcinoma of the right side of the bowel differ from that of the left?

12. What are the symptoms of intestinal obstruction?

13. What are the extra-abdominal causes of acute abdominal pain?

ANSWERS

1. **Dysphagia** may be due to abnormalities of the wall or the lumen of the oesophagus, or extrinsic pressure. Strictures of the wall include benign and malignant neoplasms, acute and chronic oesophagitis, Crohn's disease, post-radiotherapy, oesophageal diverticula and scleroderma. Abnormal contracture occurs in achalasia, abnormal relaxation of cricopharyngeus and Chagas' disease. Abnormalities within the lumen include foreign bodies and webs. Extrinsic pressure can be from a goitre, pharyngeal pouch, aortic aneurysm or abnormal aortic arch vessels, mediastinal tumours and a paraoesophageal hiatus hernia.

   Hepatomegaly: (a) infection (hepatitis A, B, C, D and E, infectious mononucleosis, hydatid cysts, amoeba, schistosomiasis and bacterial abscesses, cholangitis and portal pyaemia); (b) cellular proliferation (leukaemias, lymphoma, polycythaemia); (c) cellular infiltrates (amyloid, sarcoid); (d) metabolic (haemochromatosis, Wilson's disease, galactosaemia and drugs); (d) space-occupying lesions (abscesses, cysts, syphilitic gumma, haemangioma, hepatoma, cholangiocarcinoma, metastatic disease); (e) congestive heart failure and Budd–Chiari syndrome.

   Splenomegaly: (a) infection (viral, infective mononucleosis, typhoid, typhus, TB, septicaemic abscess, syphilis, leptospirosis, malaria, schistosomiasis, trypanosomiasis, tropical splenomegaly, hydatid cyst and kala-azar); (b) cellular proliferation (leukaemia, myelofibrosis, polycythaemia rubra vera, pernicious anaemia, hereditary spherocytosis, thalassaemia, sickle cell disease, idiopathic thrombocytopenic purpura, collagen diseases, Felty syndrome and Still's disease); (c) cellular infiltrates and metabolic (amyloid, Gaucher's disease, porphyria); (d) space-occupying lesions (cysts, angioma, lymphoma); (e) circulatory (congestion and portal hypertension, hepatic vein obstruction, right-sided heart failure, embolic infarction, splenic artery infarction and venous thromboses).

   Hepatosplemomegaly causes can be determined from the overlap of the previous two lists.

   Jaundice may be due to pre-hepatic causes (haemolytic: hereditary spherocytosis, hypersplenism), hepatic causes (liver dysfunction: hepatitis, cirrhosis, Gilbert's disease) and post-hepatic causes (obstruction to the biliary tree caused by gallstones, benign and malignant strictures, sclerosing cholangiitis, extrinsic neoplasms in the porta hepatis and head of pancreas).

Change in bowel habit: this is commonly experienced in relation to dietary changes, alcohol intake, overseas trips and changes in daily routines such as mobility, confinement to bed and in pregnancy. However, when there is an obvious cause it must be fully investigated because it is a cardinal sign of neoplasia in the older age group, as well as the other pathologies listed in the subsequent two items.

Diarrhoea: commonly infective in origin; in temperate climates, *Salmonella* and *Escherichia* spp. are common whereas in tropical areas a wide variety of bacteria, viral and parasitic agents may be involved. Other causes include: ingestion of purgatives and antibiotics, chronic pancreatitis, cystic fibrosis, small-gut abnormalities (eg gluten-induced or protein-losing enteropathy), inflammatory bowel disease (see below), surgical intervention (gastrectomy, vagotomy, blind-loop syndrome, small-gut resection, stomas), fistulae and systemic diseases (thyrotoxicosis, uraemia, carcinoid and Zollinger–Ellison syndrome). Spurious diarrhoea is the leakage of faecal fluid around impacted faeces.

Constipation is a cardinal sign of acute intestinal obstruction (see below). In these cases there is absolute constipation with no passage of flatus. Other causes include weight loss (starvation cachexia and malignant lesions), peritoneal and inflammatory disorders (appendicitis, pelvic inflammatory disease, peritonitis, perforation), biliary and renal colic, drugs (eg analgesics, ganglion blockers), adynamic bowel (Hirschsprung's and Chagas' diseases), spinal cord abnormalities, myxoedema, pelvic masses (pregnancy, fibroids, uterine and ovarian tumours) and painful lesions inhibiting defecation (abscesses and complicated haemorrhoids).

Haematemesis and melaena: melaena is the name for the black stool resulting from the digestion of blood from luminal bleeding in the upper intestinal tract. When this bleeding is profuse and from the proximal duodenum and above, it may be vomited as haematemesis. Thus, haematemesis and melaena have a common aetiology above this level. **Oesophageal bleeding** must be differentiated from haemoptysis and can result from most of the inflammatory and neoplastic causes of dysphagia listed above. Other causes of oesophageal bleeding include trauma after endoscopy, ingestion of foreign bodies and vomiting leading to tearing of the mucosa at the oesophageal junction (Mallory–Weiss tear). Some of the most severe bleeding is from oesophageal varices in liver failure and fatal bleeding occurs when an aortic aneurysm erodes into the oesophagus. Gastroduodenal haematemesis is usually due to peptic ulceration but may be caused by multiple gastric erosions and benign and malignant neoplasms. In the small gut, ectopic gastric mucosa may be present in Meckel's diverticulum or duplicated gut, causing melaena. Aortoduodenal fistulae and fistulae from infected prosthetic arterial grafts in the abdomen can also cause melaena.

Bleeding per rectum: may be overt or covert. Covert bleeding is associated with anaemia and usually originates from lesions in the right colon, which is more capacious than the left colon and therefore rarely becomes obstructed. The most common cause of overt bleeding is piles. Other causes include fistulae, fissures and any neoplasm of the colon, rectum or anal canal. Bleeding from inflammatory lesions can be more prominent than from neoplasia. Catastrophic bleeding occasionally occurs from a diverticulum. Although upper alimentary bleeding usually presents as melaena, copious bleeding may pass through the bowel with little such change. Vascular malformations can give rise to severe haemorrhage.

Obstruction: in children may be related to atresia along the length of the gut (oesophageal, pyloric, small gut, Hirschsprung's disease and imperforate anus, duodenal or Ladd's bands, annular pancreas, meconium ileus, midgut volvulus, strangulated hernias and intussusception. Adult obstruction may result from adynamic or dynamic causes. **Adynamic causes** include paralytic ileus, acute ischaemia, megacolon and Hirschsprung's and Chagas' diseases and pseudo-obstruction. **Dynamic causes** include lesions of the wall, lesions within the lumen and external compression. Lesions within the gut wall include diverticular disease, inflammatory bowel disease, carcinoma and anastomotic strictures. Luminal obstruction may be due to faecal impaction and gallstone ileus. The most common causes of external compression are adhesions and hernias. Other causes of external compression include volvulus, bands and the spread of neoplasia throughout the peritoneum and pelvis.

Pruritis ani is caused by excess sweating and poor local hygiene, skin conditions (eczema, contact dermatitis, allergy, psoriasis, lichen planus), infective lesions (sexually transmitted infections, fungal, scabies, lice, threadworms, *Candida* spp., *Trichomonas* spp.). **Other** causes include anal pathology (piles, fissures, fistulae, warts and pilus adenomas, solitary ulcers and other anal neoplasms), diarrhoea/ incontinence (sphincter malfunction, rectal prolapse, leakage of liquid paraffin), generalised causes of itching (obstructive jaundice, diabetes mellitus, hypoparathyroidism, myeloproliferative disorders and lymphomas) and psychological causes. In **babies**, pruritis ani is most commonly due to nappy rash as a result of infrequent changes and reaction to local applications.

2. **Abdominal tenderness** results from pressure over an area of inflamed parietal peritoneum. Pressure at such sites may produce voluntary contraction (**guarding**) of the lower abdominal wall. When peritonitis is present (see below), there is involuntary contraction of the muscles, producing **rigidity**. Paradoxically, the board-like rigidity seen in acute pancreatitis and perforated peptic ulcer is not associated with abdominal tenderness, because the wall is too rigid to allow deeper palpitation. When there is deeply seated or mild inflammation, superficial palpation may not produce tenderness but rapid release from deep palpation produces **rebound tenderness**. This test must, however, never be performed when tenderness has already been established because it may lead to severe pain. **Percussion rebound** is a very valuable test because, gently performed, it can localise the point of maximal involvement, eg in childhood appendicitis.

3. **Peritonism and peritonitis** are signs of peritoneal inflammation and are accompanied by marked guarding and often rigidity. Peritoneal inflammation may result from infective or non-infective causes, leading to peritonitis and peritonism respectively. Uninfected peritonism may be due to leakage of five irritant fluids (gastric or pancreatic juice, bile, urine and blood) as a result of perforation of a peptic ulcer or gallbladder, acute pancreatitis or bleeding from a ruptured ectopic pregnancy. If left untreated, these conditions progress to acute peritonitis due to secondary infection from transmural migration of gut organisms. Primary blood-borne peritonitis is secondary to bacteria from the lower bowel.

4. **Gallstones** may present with indigestion. Inflammation can cause tenderness (cholecystitis). Impaction of a gallstone in the cystic gut can cause biliary colic or a mucocele that may subsequently perforate. Stones in the common bowel duct may produce ascending cholangitis

and intermittent or progressive jaundice. They may also erode through into an adjacent small bowel and cause small-bowel obstruction.

5. **Pancreatic carcinomas** are usually slow growing. There is often vague, deep abdominal or back pain. Diagnosis may be late, when they have already invaded adjacent structures, such as the large vessels, spleen and the lesser sac. Carcinomas of the head, however, may involve the common bowel duct and investigation of the resulting progressive jaundice results in an earlier diagnosis.

6. **Diverticulosis** is a common condition in the western world, arising through a diet low in roughage and high in refined foods. Over half the population over the age of 50 are affected. **Diverticulitis** indicates a superadded infection.

7. Symptoms of **diverticular disease** include alteration in bowel habit, pain and tenderness in the left iliac fossa, and rectal bleeding that may be severe. Diverticular disease may also present with an abscess and a palpable mass in the left iliac fossa, perforation, peritonitis and sepsis. Fistulae into the bladder cause pneumaturia. Isolated diverticula in the caecum may present with a mass and are an important differential diagnosis for neoplasia.

8/9.

Crohn's disease and ulcerative colitis collectively are termed **'inflammatory bowel disease'** and may cause intrinsic or extrinsic lesions. The gut lesions (colitis) is primarily ulceration of the mucosa and submucosa of the colon and rectum. Long term, the lesions are prone to malignant change. **Crohn's disease** is associated with full-thickness inflammation of the gut wall with fissuring and skip lesions, and mainly involves the small bowel, but also the large bowel and the perianal region and can involve the entire gastro-intestinal tract. It typically involves adjacent structures such as the gut, urinary tract, vagina and skin. **Ulcerative colitis** is associated with prominent diarrhoea and occasionally fulminating toxic megacolon.

Extraintestinal manifestations of **inflammatory bowel disease** include haematological disorders (iron-deficiency and haemolytic anaemia, leukocytosis and thrombocytosis and deep vein thrombosis), skin disorders (erythema nodosum, pyoderma gangrenosa, drug reactions of erythema multiforme and finger clubbing), ocular disorders (iritis, uveitis, episcleritis, superficial keratitis with blepharitis, retinitis, retrobulbar neuritis), hepatic disease (sclerosing cholangitis, pericholangitis, fatty infiltration, cholelithiasis), renal disease (immune-mediated pyelonephritis, nephrolithiasis, glomerular nephritis, hypokalaemic nephritis) and arthropathy (ankylosing spondylitis, sacroiliitis, migratory monoarthropathy, peripheral arthritis in children).

10. Dukes' A: neoplasm confined to gut wall; Dukes' B: spread through gut wall; Dukes' C: nodal involvement. Later subclassifications included Dukes' C1 and C2, referring to the involvement of nodes around the inferior mesenteric artery, and Dukes' D for metastatic spread.

11. Lesions of the capacious right colon where faecal material is more fluid usually present with anaemia. Lesions of the left colon may present with an alteration in bowel habit and/or obstruction. Both may present with a palpable mass or spread to the adjacent peritoneum, leading to an inflammatory mass or perforation. Both may also present with signs of secondary spread to the liver.

12. The **features of intestinal obstruction** are colicky abdominal pain, vomiting, abdominal distension and absolute constipation.

13. **Extra-abdominal causes of acute abdominal pain** are often non-surgical in origin and must always be considered in the differential diagnosis of the acute abdomen. Cardinal signs are the absence of percussion or deep rebound tenderness during abdominal examination. Causes include ischaemic heart disease, pleuritic irritation from underlying lung disease, somatic nerve and root pain from herpes zoster infection, other causes of spinal root irritation (eg degenerative disease of the thoracic spine and tumours and abscesses in the thoracic spinal cord), diabetic crises, hyperparathyroidism, hyperlipidaemia, porphyria, lead colic, sickle cell crises, tabes dorsalis and Munchausen syndrome.

Lump in the groin

THE HISTORY

Hernias and groin lumps are very popular short and OSCE cases. After examining a hernia, you may be instructed to ask the patient some additional questions. Structure them as follows.

The lump itself

See page 41.

Predisposing causes

- Do you have a chronic cough/asthma/bronchitis?

- Do you do much heavy lifting?

- Do you have to strain to pass a motion? (Note that this can occur with both constipation and diarrhoea.)

- Do you have difficulty passing water?

Potential complications (strangulation and obstruction)

- Does the lump become tender or painful?

- Do you have any abdominal pain?

- Have you vomited recently?

- Have you noticed your abdomen swelling/your clothes getting tighter?

- Are you constipated?

THE EXAMINATION

In a short case, you may be asked specifically to 'examine this hernia' or 'this scrotal lump', in which case you should examine as for any lump (pages 41–43) plus perform the additional assessment outlined below. If you are asked to 'examine the groin', follow the whole examination scheme.

Note the following points:

- You may see an inguinal lump that you are certain is a hernia. However, always examine the scrotum as well. There might be dual pathology.

- Always examine both sides: 20% of hernias are bilateral.

- Try to distinguish between a direct and an indirect inguinal hernia. Some say that this is unimportant because it does not affect the patient's management. However, you cannot be faulted for being too thorough.

'Examine this patient's groin'

ACTION	NOTE
Introduce yourself	
Say what you wish to do	
Ask the patient's permission to proceed	If there is an *obvious* inguinoscrotal swelling, do not stand the patient up. Otherwise, examine with the patient standing
Expose the groin and external genitalia	

Examination for hernias

ACTION	NOTE
Stand to one side of the patient, who should be standing	If no swelling is seen, place your hand over the superficial ring (just above and medial to the pubic tubercle)
Locate the pubic tubercle	*?inguinoscrotal*
Place one hand behind patient and the examining hand over the swelling	
ASSESS THE SWELLING	
Define its characteristics (see pages 41–43)	*?size*
Superomedial to pubic tubercle inguinal hernia	*?shape*
	?fluctuant
Inferolateral to pubic tubercle femoral hernia	*?transilluminable*
Press firmly over the swelling/ superficial ring	
Ask patient to turn his or her head away from you and cough	*?expansile cough impulse*
Ask patient to try to reduce the hernia	He or she may ask to lie down to do this
While the hernia is still reduced, place two fingers over the deep ring (halfway between pubic tubercle and ASIS)	
Ask patient to cough	
Watch	
Release the pressure	*?hernia controlled by pressure over deep ring* (indicates indirect hernia)
Go to the other side of patient	
Repeat the examination	
For scrotal examination (see page 139)	

ACTION	NOTE
COMPLETE THE EXAMINATION	
Cover the patient up	
Turn to the examiner	
Ask to wash your hands	
Present your findings	

TYPICAL CASES

INGUINAL SWELLINGS AND HERNIAS

One way to remember the differential diagnosis of lumps in the groin is to think of the structures that normally lie in the region.

a. Hernias

- Inguinal (direct, indirect)
- Femoral.

b. Vascular structures

- Saphena varix
- Femoral aneurysm.

c. Lymph nodes

- Lymphadenopathy.

d. Muscle

- Psoas abscess.

e. Hip joint

- Psoas bursa.

f. Testis

- Ectopic testis (in superficial inguinal pouch)
- Undescended testis (as it emerges from superficial ring).

g. Spermatic cord

- Lipoma of the cord
- Hydrocele of the cord.

Have a clear picture of the relationship of these structures to the inguinal ligament.

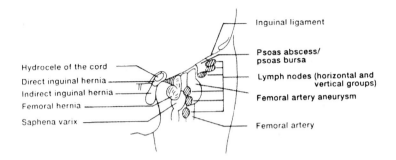

You may be asked what is meant by the term 'hernia'. The definition should roll off your tongue:

'The protrusion of the whole or part of a viscus, from its normal position, through an opening in the wall of its containing cavity.'

Another common question is: 'Why must a hernia be repaired?'

The answer is because of the potential complications of *obstruction* and *strangulation*. You should understand exactly what is meant by these two terms.

Obstruction: constriction at the neck of a hernial sac leads to obstruction of the loops of bowel within it.

Strangulation: constriction prevents venous return, causing venous congestion, arterial occlusion and gangrene. This can lead to perforation, causing peritonitis or a groin abscess.

Note that strangulation can occur without obstruction if only one wall of a viscus pouches into the sac ('Richter's hernia').

Case 1: inguinal hernia

There is not much anatomy that you need to know for finals.

However, a favourite question is to describe the anatomy of the inguinal canal: this is an intermuscular oblique passage, 4-cm long. The following structures pass through it:

- Spermatic cord/round ligament

- Ilioinguinal nerve.

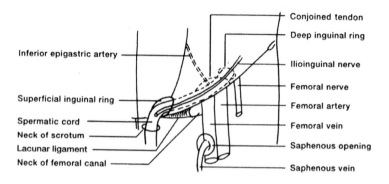

a. The walls

	Anterior	Posterior	Floor	Roof
Medially	External oblique	Conjoined tendon	Inguinal ligament + lacunar ligament	Conjoined tendon
Laterally	External + internal oblique	Fascia transversalis	Inguinal ligament	

b. The rings

External ring

This is formed by the two crura of the external oblique aponeurosis (ie it is an opening in the external oblique). It lies just above and medial to the pubic tubercle.

Internal ring

This is a U-shaped condensation of the fascia transversalis (ie it is an opening in the fascia transversalis).

It lies just above the midpoint of the inguinal ligament. The inferior epigastric artery (branch of external iliac) runs *medially*.

Note the difference between the *midpoint of the inguinal ligament* (halfway between the ASIS and the pubic tubercle) and the *midinguinal point* (halfway between the ASIS and the pubic symphysis – landmark of the femoral pulse). The midpoint of the inguinal ligament lies 1–1.5 cm lateral to the midinguinal point.

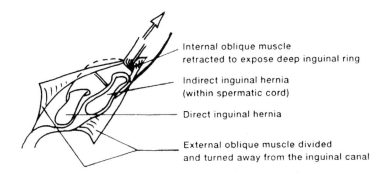

Internal oblique muscle retracted to expose deep inguinal ring

Indirect inguinal hernia (within spermatic cord)

Direct inguinal hernia

External oblique muscle divided and turned away from the inguinal canal

Understand the anatomy of direct and indirect hernias:

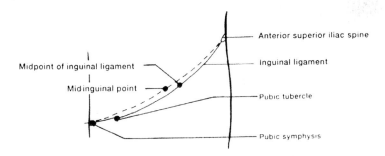

Anterior superior iliac spine

Inguinal ligament

Midpoint of inguinal ligament

Midinguinal point

Pubic tubercle

Pubic symphysis

Some examiners are keen for you to be able to distinguish clinically between a direct and an indirect hernia:

	Direct	Indirect
Extends to scrotum?	No	Yes
Direction of reduction	Straight back	Up and lateral
Controlled by pressure over internal ring?	No	Yes
Direction of reappearance after reduction	Outwards to original position	Down and medial

Treatment: surgical repair: herniotomy (removal of sac) in the neonate and herniorrhaphy (plus repair defect) in children and adults. Initial attempts are made to reduce hernias that are not tender or accompanied by systemic problems, but obstruction and strangulation are treated as an emergency.

Surgical repair can be:

1. Open repair with mesh repair.

2. Laparoscopic repair in recurrent or bilateral hernias. Two techniques are commonly used: TAPP (transabdominal preperitoneal) and TEP (total extraperitoneal) approaches.

Case 2: femoral hernia

You should know how to distinguish a femoral from an inguinal hernia clinically.

	Inguinal hernia	Femoral hernia
Position relative to pubic tubercle	Superior and medial	Inferior and lateral[a]
Palpation	Soft	Firm: like bouncing a ball underwater
Percussion	May be resonant	Dull
Auscultation	Bowel sounds commonly heard	Bowel sounds rarely heard

[a]A femoral hernia may bulge up into the groin crease (as shown on page 130).

Note the following additional points:

- In both men and women inguinal hernias are more common than femoral hernias. However, femoral hernias are more common in females than in males.

- A femoral hernia is more likely to obstruct and strangulate than an inguinal hernia because of the narrow femoral ring. Furthermore, a femoral hernia is more likely than an inguinal hernia to strangulate without obstructing (Richter's hernia).

Revise the anatomy of the neck of the femoral canal:

- Medially: lacunar ligament

- Laterally: femoral vein

- Superoanteriorly: inguinal ligament

- Inferoposterior: pectineal ligament of Astley Cooper over horizontal ramus of the pubis.

Treatment: femoral hernias have a narrow neck and are particularly prone to strangulation, possibly of the Richter variety. They therefore require early surgery and complications should be treated as an emergency. After inspecting the contents of the sac, ligating its neck and removing excess, repair is by suture of the inguinal ligament to the pectineal ligament, the fibres of which run along the superior ramus of the pubis. Two or three sutures are placed with a J-shaped needle and ligated from medial to lateral to ensure that the femoral vein is neither damaged nor compressed.

The table below summarises the clinical features of some other inguinal swellings (Cases 3–6).

	Consistency	Compressibility?	Cough impulse?	Other features
Case 3: saphena varix	Very soft	Yes	Yes	• Fluid thrill • Varicose veins
Case 4: femoral aneurysm	Firm	No	No	• Expansile pulsation • Bruit
Case 5: lymph node	Hard	No	No	• *Multiple nodules* • *Generalised lymphaden-opathy*

	Consist-ency	Compress-ibility?	Cough impulse?	Other features
Case 6: *psoas abscess*	Soft	Yes	No	• Fluctuation between parts of abscess above and below inguinal ligament

Treatment:

Case 3

A saphena varix is treated as part of varicose vein excision in symptomatic patients.

Case 4

Femoral aneurysm is treated by surgical resection and replacement with a synthetic tube (graft) oral endovascular approach.

Case 5

Lymph nodes may be part of a generalised infection. In localised infection the source must be identified and treated. Tuberculous nodes require treatment with a full course of antituberculous therapy. Primary and secondary malignant nodes require a tissue diagnosis. This might be possible through fine-needle aspiration, a full search being undertaken to identify a primary site, so that treatment of primary and secondaries can be planned.

Case 6

Psoas abscesses are drained and appropriate antituberculous therapy initiated.

FAQS AND POPULAR VIVA QUESTIONS

1. Define 'hernia'.

2. Where might you find a hernia, other than the groin?

3. What anatomical factors can predispose to inguinal hernias?

4. What are the surface markings of the superficial inguinal ring/the deep inguinal ring?

5. Describe the anatomy of the inguinal canal.

6. Describe the anatomy of the femoral canal.

7. Why do we repair hernias?

8. What are the complications of hernias?

9. What is the difference between an indirect and a direct inguinal hernia?

10. Define the terms 'herniotomy' and 'herniorrhaphy'.

11. What is the treatment of a strangulated inguinal hernia?

ANSWERS

1. A protrusion of the whole or part of a viscus from its normal position, through an opening in the wall of its containing cavity.

2. (a) **Lumbar hernia:** through a defect in the lateral abdominal wall, above the iliac crest between the posterior border of external oblique and the anterior border of latissimus dorsi. (b) **Umbilical hernia:** through a congenital defect in the umbilicus. (c) **Paraumbilical hernia:** through the linea alba, adjacent to the umbilicus. (d) **Incisional hernia:** through an old incision. (e) **Spigelian hernia:** through a defect in the lateral border of the rectus sheath, usually just below the umbilicus. (f) **Internal abdominal hernias:** through the oesophageal hiatus and other diaphragmatic congenital openings.

3. Indirect: congenital persistence of the processus vaginalis within the spermatic cord and along the inguinal canal into the scrotum. Direct: weakness in the transversalis fascia, below the conjoined tendon, bulging into the posterior aspect of the inguinal canal, medial to the inferior epigastric vessels and passing laterally alongside the spermatic cord through the superficial inguinal ring.

4. The **superficial inguinal ring** is situated above and medial to the pubic tubercle and is an opening in the external oblique aponeurosis. The **deep inguinal ring** is situated just above the midpoint of the inguinal ligament and is an opening in the transversalis fascia.

5. The **inguinal canal** extends from the deep to the superficial inguinal rings as described in (4). Posterior relations: the transversalis facia and medially conjoined tendon and inferior epigastric vessels passing upwards and medially on the tranversalis fascia. Anterior relations: the external oblique and laterally the internal oblique. Inferior relations: the inguinal ligament and medially the lacunar reflection of the inguinal ligament. The internal oblique arches over the canal to become the conjoined tendon.

6. The neck of the **femoral canal** is situated lateral to the lacunar ligament, medial to the femoral vein, with the inguinal ligament anteriorly and the superior pubic ramus posteriorly. The canal passes downwards beneath the fascia lata to the saphenous opening. Hernias pass along this pathway and through the opening, alongside the vein. As a result of the attachment of the superficial facia to the inferior

margin of the saphenous opening, femoral hernias are then directed upwards anterior to the inguinal ligament in the groin.

7/8.

Two serious **complications of hernias** are obstruction and strangulation. In obstruction, constriction of the neck of the sac leads to obstruction of the loops of small bowel within it. In strangulation, constriction of the venous return leads to congestion, arterial occlusion and gangrene, with the potential of perforation, causing peritonitis or a groin abscess. In Richter's hernia, a bulge of one wall of the viscus into the hernial sac may become strangulated without producing obstruction of the involved bowel loop.

9. An indirect hernia passes along the inguinal canal within the spermatic cord and its congenital defect. A direct inguinal hernia is through a weakness of the transversalis facia in the posterior wall, the hernial sac passing medially through the superficial inguinal ring alongside the spermatic cord.

10. **Herniotomy** involves the opening of the hernial sac, the inspection of its contents, their replacement within the abdominal wall, ligation of the neck and removal of excess tissues. In **herniorrhaphy**, there is additional repair of the abdominal wall defect. In children, where the superficial and deep inguinal rings almost overlap, a herniorrhaphy is unnecessary because, in the subsequent development of the inguinal canal, the external and internal oblique muscles come to overlay the herniotomy site.

11. An incision is made over the strangulated loop of gut, the sac is opened, infected peritoneal fluid is evacuated, and the strangulated loop is examined to assess its viability and the need for resection. Care must be taken not to lose a strangulated loop or strangulated side wall of bowel back into the abdomen without it being fully examined. If there is any doubt about this happening, or if the resection cannot be carried out through the hernial sac, a separate laparotomy incision is also required.

Urology

Urological cases present in the clinical with renal (page 109) and scrotal swellings (page 127); malignancy and infection of the renal tract and prostatic problems are not commonly associated with other abnormal physical signs. You should, however, be able to take a urological history, and know about the symptoms of prostatism and urinary tract infection, and the management of urinary catheters.

The presenting symptoms are as follows:

- Prostatism: hesitancy, frequency, poor urinary stream, terminal dribbling, incomplete evacuation, double micturition (particularly first thing in the morning), urgency, nocturia

- Frequency: note the number of times that the bladder is emptied during the day and night (D/N)

- Nocturia: the number of times getting out of bed to pass water

- Cloudy/offensive urine: infection and stagnation (obstruction, atonia)

- Dysuria: pain on passing urine – usually infection and burning or stinging

- Urgency/incontinence: usually infection, may be prostatic enlargement; stress incontinence (on coughing, laughing) usually gynaecological

- Stangury: sudden painful cessation of micturition – usually caused by vesical or urethral calculi

- Fever/systemic disturbance: infection and malignancy

- Abdominal pain: suprapubic – usually cystitis; renal colic, loin radiating to groin – calculi; loin – renal disease

- Haematuria: start, mixed or end of stream/frank blood; painful – usually infection; painless – malignancy must be excluded

- Polyuria: passing large volumes of urine – increased intake, diabetes mellitus/insipidus

- Sexual history: orientation, contacts.

Examination includes looking for nephrectomy and suprapubic scars (see page 105); the loins for renal masses (see page 113, Cases 8 and 10, and page 147, answer 1); the iliac fossae for transplanted kidneys (see page 114, Case 11, and page 148, answer 5); and the scrotum (see below): tell the examiner that you would always add a rectal examination in your clinical practice. A general examination (see page 9) is an essential part of the assessment of all renal disease and malignancies of the renal tract, because there might be abnormal systemic signs (at the end ask for dipstick).

Examination of the external genitalia

LOOK	
Observe the anterior aspect of the scrotum	skin: *?colour*
	swelling: *?inguinal, ?scrotal*
Observe the posterior aspect of the scrotum, pulling on posterior skin, **not** the testes	
Penis	*?circumscribed*
	?retractable foreskin
	?balanitis
	?meatal discharge
FEEL (?gloves provided)	
Roll the testes *gently* between your thumb (in front) and index finger (behind)	*?both testes palpable*
Locate the epididymis (above and posterior to testis)	*?epididymal swelling*
Feel along the spermatic cord	*?cord swelling*

ASSESSMENT OF SWELLING

Try to locate its upper edge	*?can you get above it*
Define its characteristics (see pages 41–43)	*?size*
	?shape
	?surface
	?consistency
	?fluctuant
	?transilluminable
Try to feel testis	*?testis separate from swelling*

COMPLETE THE EXAMINATION

Cover the patient up

Turn to the examiner

Ask to wash your hands

Present your findings

Case 1: suprapubic mass

Suprapubic masses are easily missed. The two characteristics of a pelvic swelling are:

1. Cannot get below it.

2. May be palpated bimanually on vaginal or rectal examination.

The most common cause is an enlarged bladder. This has the following characteristics:

- Dull to percussion

- Fluid thrill

- Direct pressure produces desire to micturate.

In the female, do not forget obstetric and gynaecological causes: the most frequent pelvic mass in the female is the pregnant uterus. Also consider a large ovarian cyst and uterine fibroids.

Manual examination improves diagnosis of obstetric and gynaecological causes.

Treatment: an enlarged bladder usually requires decompression by transurethral or suprapubic catheterisation. Emergency surgery may be required for ectopic pregnancies and complications of ovarian cysts. As much ovarian tissue as possible is preserved in the premenstrual years, but ovarian cancer requires extensive clearance, as well as a chemotherapeutic approach. Uterine cancer, fibroids and other lesions may require hysterectomy with or without oophorectomy.

SCROTAL AND INGUINOSCROTAL SWELLINGS

It is unlikely that you will be given a patient with a very tender swelling in an examination because this usually implies the following:

- Torsion of the testis: a surgical emergency

- Severe epididymo-orchitis: rare.

A simplified diagnostic flowchart that excludes the latter two conditions is given below.

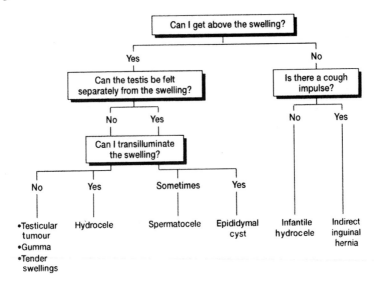

Case 1: testicular tumour

This is an opaque mass, not felt discretely from the testis. It is usually painless but occasionally causes a dull ache. There is usually loss of sensation in the mass.

Remember that it may be associated with a secondary hydrocele.

Note that lymphatic spread is along the site of its embryological origin, ie to para-aortic lymph nodes. It spreads to inguinal nodes only if the scrotum is invaded.

Investigation: the initial diagnosis is a clinical one. Tumour markers may be elevated – β human chorionic gonadotropin (90% in teratoma, 25% in seminoma), α-fetoprotein (50% in teratoma) plus alkaline phosphatase (50% in seminoma). CT is undertaken to identify para-aortic or mediastinal lymph nodes or secondaries in the liver or lungs.

Treatment: orchidectomy via an inguinal approach. The testis is delivered through the incision in the external oblique and a vascular clamp applied to the spermatic cord, while a biopsy and frozen section are taken to confirm the diagnosis. A high ligation of the cord and orchidectomy are undertaken. Subsequent management depends on the stage and the pathology:

Stage 1: rising tumour markers post-orchidectomy

Stage 2: abdominal nodes

Stage 3: supradiaphragmatic nodes

Stage 4: lung or liver metastases.

The subsequent treatment of testicular seminomas is radiotherapy for stages 1 and 2, combination chemotherapy for stage 2 if nodes are >5 cm and for cysts after radiotherapy, and for stages 3 and 4.

In teratoma, surgical resection of abdominal nodes is advocated as well as combination chemotherapy. Testicular lymphomas are treated by orchidectomy and chemotherapy.

Case 2: varicocele

This is a dilatation and elongation of the pampiniform plexus of veins, usually found on the left.

It feels like a 'bag of worms', and may have a cough impulse.

It can only be felt with the patient standing.

Recent onset of a left-sided varicocele in an older man may be associated with a left renal cell carcinoma which is invading the left renal vein, thus occluding the left testicular vein.

Treatment: in symptomatic enlargement of the pampiniform plexus and in the management of infertility the plexus is excised, preserving the testicular vein within the spermatic sheath, using an inguinal incision. Current options also include endovascular coiling of the varicocele.

Case 3: hydrocele

This is a swelling that cannot be felt separately from the testis. It is fluctuant and transilluminable. It is due to excessive fluid collecting in the tunica vaginalis.

Understand the anatomy of the four types of hydrocele. All of these come into your differential diagnosis of inguinal and inguinoscrotal lumps. A vaginal hydrocele is by far the most common. The features of the four types of hydrocele are summarised in the table overleaf.

Treatment: the hydrocele may be secondary to trauma (haematocele), infection or a tumour. Idiopathic hydroceles can be managed conservatively. Aspiration is possible although recurrence is usual. Definitive treatment is by surgical excision of the tunica vaginalis or incision of the sac and radial plication sutures from within it to reduce its size.

Type	Age	Communication with peritoneal cavity?	Note	Diagram
Vaginal	All	No	May be *secondary* to underlying infection or a testicular tumour	
Congenital	Child (aged <3 years)	Yes	Main differential diagnosis is an indirect inguinal hernia: communicating orifice is too small for hernia to develop	
Infantile	All	No	Due to incomplete reabsorption of fluid from the tunica vaginalis after the processus vaginalis seals off	
Encysted hydrocele of the cord	All	No	May occur anywhere along the cord, causing a scrotal *or* inguinal lump	

Case 4: epididymal cyst

Similar to a hydrocele, this is brilliantly transilluminable. However, the testis can be felt separately.

Note that if it is filled with many sperm it can be opaque. In this case, it is called a *spermatocele*.

Treatment: usually conservative but cysts might be excised if they are producing symptoms; care is taken not to damage surrounding structures because this can impair fertility.

Case 5: Absent testis in a child

Put your hand just lateral to the external ring and apply firm pressure downwards and medially. If you can 'milk' the testis down into the scrotum, the testis is *retractile*: descent is normal, but excessive cremasteric muscle activity in young children leads to the testis being drawn up.

Look carefully for other swellings in the area; there may be an *ectopic* testis. You may feel a lump in the following positions:

- Superficial inguinal pouch (superficial to external oblique and lateral to the pubic tubercle)

- Femoral canal (medial thigh)

- Perianally.

Once you have *excluded* retractile and ectopic testes, you can diagnose an incompletely descended testis.

Remember to search for an inguinal hernia. This is present in 90% of cases of incompletely descended testes.

Treatment: undescended testes usually descend into the scrotum by the age of 2 years. Orchidopexy is undertaken after this age as (1) infertility is likely after puberty, (2) the testes are more likely to undergo torsion and (3) the testes have a tenfold increased incidence of malignancy. The testes may lie in the inguinal canal or just above (identification may be helped by CT). The spermatic vessels are preserved but other restricting tissues are excised to allow the testes to reach the scrotum. Ectopic testes are similarly mobilised and placed within the scrotum.

FAQS AND POPULAR VIVA QUESTIONS

1. What is the differential diagnosis for a left upper quadrant mass?

2. How do you differentiate between an enlarged spleen and an enlarged kidney?

3. What are the typical signs found in renal cell carcinoma?

4. How would you investigate and treat a patient with renal cell carcinoma?

5. What clinical signs would indicate that a patient has had a renal transplant?

6. Name three risk factors for end-stage renal failure.

7. How do you manage patients with renal transplants?

8. What are the causes of haematuria?

9. How do bladder tumours present?

10. What do you understand by benign prostatic hyperplasia?

11. A man is found to have a craggy prostate on attending the clinic with back pain – how do you proceed?

12. What is the Gleason score?

13. How would you manage a patient with a testicular tumour?

A N S W E R S

1. The **differential diagnosis for a left upper quadrant mass** includes:
   a. Renal: renal cysts, renal cancers / metastases, hydronephrosis, perinephric abscess
   b. Spleen: splenomegaly, splenic artery aneurysm
   c. Colon: colon tumour
   d. Stomach: gastric tumour.

2. Differences between a renal and a splenic mass:
   A renal mass:
   a. On palpation is ballotable
   b. On palpation has no medial notch
   c. On palpation one can 'get above it'
   d. On inspiration descends vertically down
   e. On percussion it is resonant to percussion (has overlying loops of bowel).

   An enlarged spleen:
   a. On palpation is not ballotable
   b. On palpation has a medial notch
   c. On palpation one 'cannot get above it' (upper edge is hidden by thoracic cage)
   d. On inspiration: descends diagonally towards right iliac fossa
   e. On percussion it is dull.

3. **Typical signs of a renal cell carcinoma:**
   a. Renal cell carcinoma classically presents with the triad of flank pain, flank mass and haematuria. In reality these three symptoms rarely occur together.
   b. The presence of a left testicular varicocele indicates tumour spread in the left renal vein with obstruction of the left testicular / gonadal vein, giving rise to the varicocele.
   c. Hypertension can occur due to excess renin secretion by the tumour. This exemplifies a paraneoplastic syndrome. Hypercalcaemia may also be detected.
   d. Bedside urine analysis may reveal haematuria.

4. **Investigation for a renal cell carcinoma:**
Investigation includes renal ultrasound and contrast CT of the chest, abdomen and pelvis for staging.
Treatment for renal cell carcinoma is radical nephrectomy. Small lesions under 4 cm may be amenable to partial nephrectomy. Radiation and chemotherapy have poor results. Immunotherapy requires further investigation, although it has produced encouraging results in select patient groups.

5. **Clinical signs of renal transplantation:**
   a. A non-tender mass in the iliac fossa (the transplanted kidney) with an overlying J-shaped incision (Rutherford Morison scar)
   b. A forearm or cubital fossa scar indicating a previous reversal of an arteriovenous fistula used for dialysis
   c. Evidence of Cushing syndrome secondary to chronic steroid use for immunosupression (see page 36).

6. **Three risk factors for end-stage renal failure:**
   a. Hypertension
   b. Diabetes mellitus
   c. Polycystic renal disease.

7. **Management of patients with a renal transplant:**
Patients with renal transplants need to be on life-long immuno-suppressive therapy, avoid nephrotoxic agents (eg NSAIDs) and have regular follow-up with renal physicians. They must be carefully monitored for post-transplant complications, including post-transplant ATN (acute tubular necrosis) and anastomotic urine leaks in the immediate stages, immune rejection of kidney and renal vascular thrombosis.

8. **Causes of haematuria:**
   a. Tumours: renal cell carcinomas, bladder transitional cell carcinomas, prostate adenocarcinoma
   b. Trauma: post insertion of Foley catheter, after cystoscopy or after urethral injury in pelvic fractures
   c. Infection: cystitis, prostatitis
   d. Inflammation: nephritic syndrome
   e. Mechanical: urinary stones
   f. Medical: coagulopathies
   g. 'Red herrings': ingestion of beetroot, jaundice causing dark urine.

9. **Presentation of bladder tumours:**

   Bladder tumours are difficult to diagnose clinically. Possible presentations include:

   a. Haematuria

   b. Changes in urinary stream if the tumour involves the bladder outlet

   c. Abdominal or pelvic masses associated with inguinal lymphadenopathy (rarely found in early lesions).

10. **Benign prostatic hypertrophy** is an enlargement of the prostate gland, affecting mostly the transitional and peri-urethral zones.

    This can cause partial or complete urinary obstruction, manifested as a weak urinary stream, urinary frequency, nocturia, dribbling, a feeling of incomplete bladder emptying and urinary retention.

    It commonly affects men over the age of 60.

    Digital rectal examination reveals a smooth but enlarged prostate gland. Transrectal ultrasonography can provide a volumetric assessment of prostate size.

    Medical management includes:

    a. Alpha-adrenergic blockers, eg tamsulosin

    b. 5-alpha reductase inhibitors, eg finasteride.

    Surgical management consists of transurethral resection of the prostate (TURP).

11. In a patient with a craggy (enlarged / irregular) prostate and back pain you have to suspect a diagnosis of **prostate cancer** with bone metastases:

    a. As for any condition take a focused history and perform a physical examination, including a digital rectal examination.

    b. The next step is to measure the level of PSA (prostate-specific antigen) which is a marker of prostate cancer.

    c. Perform other routine blood tests: LFTs for evidence of liver metastases; high ALP and calcium levels may be indicative of bone metastases.

    d. Perform a transrectal ultrasound and transrectal biopsy in order to get a tissue diagnosis.

    e. CT or MRI scan can be used to assess local and distal spread of disease (tumour staging), as well as any bone lesions.

f.   Refer for a combined urology/oncology multidisciplinary team opinion.

12. **The Gleason score** is a histological scoring system used to determine the grade of differentiation of prostate cancer. This is based on the two most common glandular patterns seen on prostate biopsy. Each of commonest patterns is scored from 1 to 5.

    The sum of the two gives an overall score out of 10. A score of 1 represents a well-differentiated tumour (best outcomes), while 10 is a very poorly differentiated one (worst outcomes).

13. In **testicular tumour** the initial diagnosis is a clinical one. Tumour markers may be elevated: β human chorionic gonadotropin (90% in teratoma, 25% seminoma), α-fetoprotein (50% in teratoma) and alkaline phosphatase (50% in seminoma). CT identifies para-aortic or mediastinal lymph nodes or secondaries in the liver or lungs. The treatment is orchidectomy via an inguinal approach. The testis is delivered through the incision in the external oblique and a vascular clamp is applied to the spermatic cord while a biopsy and frozen section are taken to confirm the diagnosis. A high ligation of the cord and orchidectomy are then undertaken. Subsequent management depends on the stage and the pathology. Stage 1: rising tumour markers post-orchidectomy; stage 2: abdominal nodes; stage 3: supradiaphragmatic nodes; and stage 4: lung or liver metastases.

Treatment of seminomas: radiotherapy for stages 1 and 2. Combination chemotherapy for stage 2 if nodes are >5 cm and for cysts after radiotherapy, and for stages 3 and 4. **Treatment of teratomas:** surgical resection of abdominal nodes as well as combination chemotherapy. **Treatment of lymphomas:** orchidectomy and chemotherapy.

13 A limb

Most of this book is devoted to specific systems or parts of the body. However, you may be asked for a more general approach (as considered on page 9), and similarly you may be told to examine a limb, with no clues from the examiner as to which system is abnormal. Always approach the problem by looking systematically and remarking on any abnormalities that you see. Then go on to examine the appropriate systems.

In the upper limb, this may focus on the hand (see page 189), or the joints of hand and the rest of the limb. In the lower limb it may relate to the joints or the vascular system, as considered in subsequent sections. The scheme on the following pages gives an initial approach to examining a leg.

'Examine this patient's leg'

ACTION	NOTE
Introduce yourself	
Say what you wish to do	
Ask the patient's permission to proceed	
Expose both legs to the groin	
LOOK	skin: *?scars; /swelling/ulcers;?varicose veins/signs of venous insufficiency* (see pages 40, 227 and 229)
If obvious joint/orthopaedic problems, you may switch to examination of the hip and knee (see pages 160, 173) and to assess the gait (see page 165): but still do not forget distal pulses and sensation	*?trophic changes/ischaemic ulceration/gangrene* (see page 217) soft tissues: *?swelling of knee* (see pages 172 and 182) *?quadriceps wasting* (see page 174) *?gluteal wasting* (see page 161)

ACTION	NOTE
	bony alignment, skin creases: *?genu varum/valgum* (see page 182)
	?disparity in leg length (see page 161)
FEEL	
Feel pulses	See page 210
Check for lymphadenopathy	*?warmth ?pitting oedema*
MOVE	
Check active and passive movement of each joint	
Feel for crepitus	
Rapid neurological assessment	Upper limb – see page 234
Test response to light touch (using cotton wool; first demonstrate with eyes open: 'Say yes every time I touch you')	
Test response to a pinprick: 'Is this sharp?'	
Look for muscle wasting and abnormal movements	
Check power, tone and reflexes	
Detailed examination of lower limb sensation and motor function	
Lower limb **sensory testing** (with eyes closed) of dermatomes:	
Touch (cotton wool): first demonstrate with eyes open: 'Say yes every time you feel me touch you'	Ll groin; L3 and L4 front of knee; L5 front of ankle (often overlap); S1 sole; S2 midline strip along back of leg; S3 buttocks (you walk on S1 and sit on S3)

ACTION	NOTE
Repeat for **pain** (sterile needle or broken end of wooden stick – 'Is this sharp?') and **temperature** (side of finger vs cold side of tuning fork, or test tubes of warm and cold water – 'Is this hot or cold?')	
Vibration – vibrating base of tuning fork on medial malleolus: 'Say when it stops'	
Position sense – recognising direction of movement – hold sides of big toe: 'This is up and this is down'	
Motor testing:	
Power – dorsiflexion and plantarflexion of foot against resistance	
Tone – passive flexion and extension of relaxed knee, clonus	
Coordination – heel up and down along opposite shin – eyes open and then closed	
Reflexes – knee L3 and L4; ankle S1 and S2 Plantar response	
Note wasting and abnormal movements	
Individual muscles – active and passive movements, and against resistance – unable to raise leg off bed with femoral nerve damage; foot drop with sciatic damage	L2-3: hip flexion L3-4: knee extension; kick the door L4: heel walking L4-5 dorsiflexion L5: dorsiflexion big toe L5-S1: knee flexion, plantar flexion, hip extension S1: tip toe S1-2: buckle my shoe

14 A joint

The most common orthopaedic long and short cases are hip and knee. However, do not panic if you are given a shoulder, an elbow, an ankle or a back to examine. Follow the same routine for all joints and with your chosen colleague (see page 5) go through the routine of look, feel, move and measure, and tell the examiner you would like a radiograph to confirm your findings. Never forget to expose both sides of the body, and at the end to check pulses and peripheral sensation. (In a rheumatological examination, you are expected to examine gait, arms, legs and spine – GALS.) Your routine should include the joint above and below.

'Examine this patient's joint'

ACTION	NOTE	
Introduce yourself		
Say what you wish to do		
Ask the patient's permission to proceed		
Expose the joints of both sides of the body		
LOOK	skin:	*?creases ?erythema*
		?rashes
		?scars
		?sinuses
	soft tissue:	*?swelling*
		?effusion, bursae
	muscle:	*?wasting*

ACTION	NOTE
	bony alignment:
	?deformity
	?valgus
	?varu
	?shortening
	?lengthening
Ask the patient if he or she has any pain	
FEEL	
Ask if there is any tenderness	
Run the back of your hand over the joint	temperature: *?warm*
Feel any swelling	swelling: *?fluid, ?fluctuant*
	?soft tissue
	?bony
Feel over the joint line	*?tenderness*
MOVE (active, passive, resisted)	In the lower limb, the gait is critical – if the patient is sitting you are probably meant to start with this
Ask patient to move the joint in each direction in turn	*?range of active movement*
Move joint in all directions, feeling for crepitus	*?range of passive movement*
	?contracture, fixed
	?crepitus, abnormal movement, instability, telescoping
	?clicks, creaks, locking
Resisted movement	*?pain, ?weakness*

ACTION	NOTE
MEASURE • range • shortening/lengthening (true/apparent)	?estimate, ?goniometer Compare lengths of proximal and distal bones on each side
• muscle wasting Examine the ankle pulses and sensation over the toe. Tell the examiner you would like to examine the joint above and below and X-ray in two planes	Compare proximal limb circumference on each side – taken at the same distances from the olecranon and tibial tubercles
Cover patient and make him or her comfortable	
Turn to examiner and say that you would like to confirm your findings with a radiograph	

POPULAR VIVA QUESTIONS

1. Describe the clinical features of a patient with osteoarthritis (OA) of the knee.

2. Which compartment of the knee is most often affected by OA?

3. How would you manage OA of the knee?

4. What features of OA would you expect to see on a joint X-ray?

5. What is the differential diagnosis of a red, hot, swollen joint?

6. How would you diagnose a red, hot, swollen joint?

7. When should you suspect septic arthritis of a joint?

8. When would you aspirate a swollen joint?

9. How would you manage gout?

10. You have finished examining a painful knee. What would you like to do next?

ANSWERS

1. The patient has an antalgic gait, with a varus deformity of the knee. On palpation of the knee joint osteophytes are present. Passive movement of the knee reveals crepitus. The quadriceps is wasted due to lack of activity secondary to pain.

2. The medial knee compartment is most often affected by osteoarthritis.

3. Initial management involves analgesia, weight loss if required, use of walking aids and physiotherapy. Osteotomy of the involved tibial compartment may be the initial therapeutic approach. Older patients or those with significant symptoms require a knee replacement.

4. Remember the mnemonic for **features of osteoarthritis on an X-ray:** LOSS

    Loss of joint space

    Osteophytes

    Subchondral cyst

    Subchondral sclerosis

5. **Differential diagnosis of a red swollen joint:**

    a. Inflammation (synovitis in rheumatoid arthritis)

    b. Degenerative cartilage damage (osteoarthritis)

    c. Crystal deposition (gout, pseudogout)

    d. Infection (septic arthritis)

    e. Trauma (haemarthrosis, meniscal tears, ligamentous injury, bone fracture, joint capsule tears).

6. **Diagnosis of a red swollen joint** requires a focused history with the above differential in mind, followed by an examination. Perform simple blood tests to looks for evidence of infection or inflammation (WBC, CRP, ESR) . Rheumatoid factor and ANA levels are requested if the history is suggestive of non-infectious inflammatory disease. Do a full set of X-rays to identify any evidence of rheumatoid or osteo-arthritic changes, as well as fractures.

    Discuss joint aspiration with your Consultant, (for crystals and culture – see question 8).

7. If the joint cannot be moved due to pain or swelling and the patient is tachycardic or has a pyrexia, consider **septic arthritis** as a diagnosis (unlikely in an examination, but an important aspect of the differential diagnosis). Also determine source of sepsis (eg superificial trauma or infection/abscess at another site causing haematogenous spread). Septic arthritis is an orthopaedic emergency. Aspirate joint, sending fluid for Gram stain and culture, but get a senior opinion first. For gout (urate crystals) or pseudogout (calcium pyrophosphate crystals) analyse aspirated fluid under polarised light microscopy.

8. **Aspiration** is necessary in three main circumstances:

    a. To diagnose the cause of a swollen joint (septic arthritis: microscopy and Gram stain; gout: crystals; trauma: blood)

    b. To relieve pain and discomfort caused by swelling (although this may only be temporary)

    c. To aspirate pus and perform a joint washout (this requires more than just a needle and syringe and so needs to be undertaken by orthopaedic surgeons in a sterile environment).

    Every time a joint capsule is breached the patient is exposed to the risk of septic arthritis. Currently many hospitals strongly discourage joint aspiration by junior doctors or performance of the procedure on the ward or in the Emergency Department, where the risk of introducing infection is high (the consequences are potentially disastrous after knee replacement).

    This can be a trick question in the examination, so always state that you would seek orthopaedic advice before considering aspirating a joint. Follow this advice once you qualify.

9. **Gout** requires NSAID analgesia (eg diclofenac) in the short term (acute episodes), followed by long-term allopurinol to reduce uric acid levels.

10. When finishing an examination say you would like to examine the joint above and the joint below (hip and ankle) to ensure that the pain doesn't radiate to the knee from other joints. Ask to examine anterior and lateral X-rays of the affected knee, as well as X-rays of the contralateral knee joint (in two planes).

15 The hip

THE HISTORY

Pain

Ask the usual questions about pain (see page 25). Be clear as to where your patient's pain is felt *maximally* and where it *radiates*. Ask specifically if there is any knee pain. When enquiring into exacerbating factors, ask about actions that load the joint, eg putting on socks, sitting in a low chair, rising from a sitting position and walking. Question the character of the pain: throbbing pain – abscess (? systemic symptoms); aching – arthritis; burning – neuralgia; stabbing – tendon or muscle rupture.

Neurological pain may be accompanied by focal or generalized muscle weakness or sensory loss.

Stiffness

Ask if this is worse in the morning, on movement or after staying in one position. Pain and swelling around the hip may indicate non-orthopaedic problems, such as a hernia (see page 129).

Walking

- Ask how far the patient can walk.

- Has he or she noticed a limp or change in leg length?

- Ask in detail about aids and appliances: does the patient need a walking stick or a Zimmer frame?

In a long case, you must take a detailed social history. Find out how the problem affects the patient's lifestyle and whether it is deteriorating. Ask about the involvement of other joints: many patients with osteoarthritis or rheumatoid arthritis of the hip will have had other joint replacements. You are unlikely to encounter a child in finals, but remember presentation may be a limp or delayed walking, as well as the above symptoms. Aetiological factors are considered in the FAQs at the end of the chapter.

THE EXAMINATION

The examination of the hip and knee is where most candidates let themselves down. You will probably not have had nearly as much practice as, say, in examining an abdomen. Practise on each other: it is very easy for the examiner to see if you have done it before.

Most of the patients in short cases will have osteoarthritis and will be fairly fragile. If they are supine when you are introduced, it is probably simpler to start examining in this position. However, never forget to stand the patient up to perform the Trendelenburg test and to watch the gait – if they are sitting, start with these manouvres.

In a long case, it is essential to examine the peripheral vascular system and to look for signs of infection in the leg. Both ischaemia and infection could potentially compromise a total hip replacement.

'Examine this patient's hip'

ACTION	NOTE
Introduce yourself	
Say what you wish to do	
Ask the patient's permission to proceed	
Expose both legs with the patient supine	
Check that the ASISs are at the same level	
STAND Look again:	
• anteriorly	*?rotational deformity*
• laterally	*?pelvic tilt, valgus, varus*
• posteriorly	*?increased lumbar lordosis, kyphosis*
	?scoliosis
	?gluteal wasting

ACTION	NOTE
a. Trendelenburg test	
Sit on a chair, facing the patient	The patient may rest his or her of hands on your shoulders to maintain balance
Place one hand on each side the patient's pelvis	
Ask the patient to stand on one leg	*?hip rises on opposite side* (negative test – normal)
Feel if the hip on the side rises or falls	*?hip falls on opposite side* (positive test – abnormal see page 166)
Repeat on the opposite side	
b. Gait	
Ask the patient to walk away from you and then towards you	*?Trendelenburg gait*
	?antalgic gait
	?ataxic gait
	?spastic gait
Watch carefully	*?supports, eg stick, frame*
LOOK	
Roll the patient to one side to observe the buttock and posterior thigh	skin: *?scars* *?sinuses*
	soft tissues: *?swelling* (the hip joint is deep and swelling is not usually seen)
	muscle: *?gluteal wasting*
Look at the ankles	bony alignment: *?obvious difference in leg length*
Look at the position of the patella and foot on each side	*?external rotation*
Look at the angle between the thigh and the bed	*?fixed flexion deformity*

ACTION	NOTE
MEASURE	If there is a fixed deformity, place unaffected leg in the same position as the affected leg
Measure from the ASIS to the medial malleolus	*?true leg lengths*
Measure from the xiphisternum to the medial malleolus	*?apparent leg lengths* (see page 167)
If there is any disparity in true leg length, ask the patient to bend the knees, keeping the ankles together	*?shortening below knee* (tibial shortening)
Compare the position of the two knees	*?shortening above knee* (femoral shortening)
If shortening is above the knee, put your thumbs on ASISs and feel down with your fingers until you reach the top of the greater trochanters	*?Is there a difference in the distance between ASIS and greater trochanter* (suggests shortening is in the hip joint itself)
FEEL	
Ask if there is any tenderness	
Palpate over greater trochanter	*?tenderness*
Palpate over anterior joint line (just lateral to femoral pulse)	Heat and swelling NB differential (see page 129)
MOVE (active, passive, resisted)	
a. Thomas' test and flexion	see page 168
Place your left hand in the hollow of the lumbar spine	
Flex the hip and knee of the unaffected side until the lumbar spine straightens	*?range of flexion of unaffected side* (normally 130°)
Look to see if hip of the affected side lifts up from the bed	*?fixed flexion deformity of affected hip*

ACTION	NOTE
Flex the hip and knee of the affected side	*?range of flexion of affected hip*
b. Abduction and adduction	
Rest your left forearm across the ASISs, keeping one hand on the pelvis	This stabilises the pelvis
Hold the ankle with the other hand	
First abduct and then adduct the leg until the pelvis starts to move	*?range of abduction* (normally 45°) *?range of adduction* (normally 30°)
c. Rotation	
Go to the end of the bed	Rotation may also be tested with the hip and knee flexed to 90°
Grasp the ankles and rotate each leg	*?range of internal and external rotation* (normally both 45°)
Watch the patellae	
COMPLETE THE EXAMINATION	
Make sure that patient is comfortable	
Turn to the examiner	
Present your findings	

TYPICAL CASES

Case 1: hip pain

If you meet a patient with a hip disorder in the long case/OSLER, he or she will almost certainly complain of pain.

You should know the characteristics of hip pain: this is usually felt maximally in the anterior groin. However, it is poorly defined and radiates variably to the following areas:

- Anterior thigh

- Lateral thigh

- Buttock

- Anterior knee

- Anterior lower leg.

Remember that a patient with a primary hip disorder can present with isolated *knee* pain. This is because both the hip and knee contribute fibres to the obturator and femoral nerves.

Use the table opposite to differentiate hip pain from other local or distant causes.

Diagnosis: by clinical examination of the joints. Also assess for sensory and motor loss suggesting nerve damage. Radiographs identify abnormalities of the spine, pelvis and hip (important to compare the two sides), and are supplemented by images that identify soft-tissue changes of the spine, pelvis and hip joint.

Treatment: this depends on identified cause of pain. Bursae can usually be treated conservatively until the inflammation subsides. Arthritic pain is managed by non-steroidal anti-inflammatory drugs, although preferably not long-term. The lateral cutaneous nerve of the thigh should be released in meralgia paraesthetica. A protruded disc and peripheral vascular stenotic problems may require surgical management. Severe hip arthritis may require prosthetic hip replacement or hip joint resurfacing. In all cases, consider physiotherapy, the use of a walking stick, and weight reduction.

	Site of maximum pain	Radiation	Exacerbating factors
Hip pain	Anterior groin	Wide and variable (see above)	See history above
Trochanteric bursitis	Greater trochanter	Lateral thigh	Lying on affected side
Meralgia paraesthetica (entrapment of lateral cutaneous nerve of thigh)	Anterolateral thigh	None	• Pregnancy • Tight corsets • Jeans
Sacroiliac pain	Deep in buttock	Posterior thigh	Standing on one leg (affected side)
Nerve root pain due to prolapsed disc	• Groin • Back	None	Straining/ coughing
Ischaemic pain due to aortoiliac disease (see page 217)	• Calf • Thigh • Buttock	None	Walking

Case 2: abnormal gait

You may be asked to describe the gait of a patient with hip pathology.

The two main types are the **antalgic (painful)** gait and the **Trendelenburg** gait (**waddling** gait if bilateral). You should know how they differ.

	Antalgic gait	Trendelenburg gait
Cause	Painful hip	Inefficient hip abduction
Weight-bearing/ stance phase	Shortened	Pelvis droops on opposite side
Direction to which body leans while weight bearing	Towards affected side	Towards unaffected side

You may be asked to describe the mechanism of the Trendelenburg gait. This is probably best understood by considering the Trendelenburg test. Normally, when standing on one leg, the abductors on the weight-bearing side contract so that the pelvis rises on the opposite side. A positive Trendelenburg test occurs when there is any inefficiency of hip abduction: the pelvis droops towards the unsupported side – the pelvis has to be raised for the swinging leg to clear the ground.

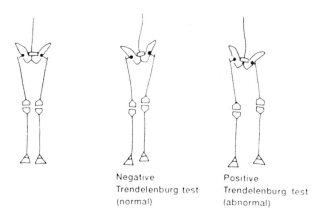

Negative
Trendelenburg test
(normal)

Positive
Trendelenburg test
(abnormal)

Inefficiency of hip abduction occurs as a result of the following factors.

a. Disturbance in the pivotal mechanism:

- dislocation or subluxation of the hip

- shortening of the femoral neck.

b. Weakness of the hip abductors (gluteus medius and minimus):

myopathy (usually bilateral): osteoarthritis; previous arthroplasty

neuropathy (L5 root lesion, usually unilateral).

Treatment: see Case 1.

Case 3: arthritis of the hip

A patient with primary osteoarthritis of the hip is a very common short or long case. You could also be given a patient with rheumatoid arthritis and you should know how to distinguish the two conditions (see page 180). A patient with osteoarthritis will complain of hip pain (see Case 1). This will initially occur only after activity, but later be present at rest. Look carefully at the gait (see Case 2).

You may be asked the reasons why you measure apparent leg length and perform Thomas' test: arthritis may result in contractures that give rise to *deformities*, and osteophytes inhibit movement. The most common are *fixed adduction and flexion deformities*. Both can be masked by compensatory movements.

The aim of measuring apparent leg length and of performing Thomas' test is to unmask these contractures.

a. Apparent leg shortening

A fixed adduction deformity tends to cross the legs. Therefore the pelvis compensates by tilting towards the affected side. This leads to apparent leg shortening. (True shortening arises from loss of joint space or arthroplasty.)

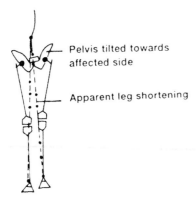

Pelvis tilted towards affected side

Apparent leg shortening

b. Thomas' test

A fixed flexion deformity can be completely masked when lying flat, by a lumbar lordosis. This is unmasked by performing Thomas' test.

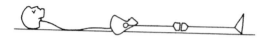

At rest, both legs rest straight on the couch, the normal lumbar lordosis masks any fixed hip flexion.

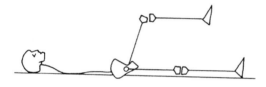

Normal – the right hip extension keeps the right leg straight and in contact with the couch

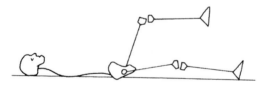

Positive Thomas test: flexion of normal left hip reveals fixed flexion of the right

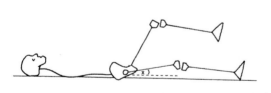

Use your right hand to flex the left leg and slide your left fingers under the back to feel when it is flat – at this point the angle x gives the amount of fixed flexion.

Treatment: see Case 1.

POPULAR VIVA QUESTIONS

1. What are the risk factors for congenital dislocation of the hip?

2. How do we screen for congenital dislocation of the hip?

3. How would you manage a baby presenting with congenital dislocation of the hip?

4. What is a slipped upper femoral epiphysis?

5. What is protrusio acetabuli?

6. What is Perthes' disease?

7. What is the difference between true and apparent leg shortening?

8. Describe the radiological appearances of osteoarthritis and rheumatoid arthritis.

9. How would you manage a patient with osteoarthritis of the hip?

10. What are the operations available for a patient with osteoarthritis of the hip?

11. What are the complications of a total hip replacement?

12. What are the contraindications to a total hip replacement?

13. Describe Garden's classification of fractured neck of femur. What is its significance?

ANSWERS

1. Developmental dysplasia **(congenital dislocation of the hip)** occurs in up to 5/1000 live deliveries. It has a polygenic inheritance pattern and is associated with high maternal relaxin and breech position of the baby. It is associated with acetabular and proximal femoral dysplasia.

2. In neonates, screen with Ortolani's test: abduction of the hips in 90° flexion is impeded; pressure on greater trochanters reduces the hips with a clunk and further movement is then possible. Barlow's

test attempts to lever the hips in and out of the acetabulum during abduction. Late features are asymmetry, clicking and difficulty in changing nappies.

3. Diagnosis is by clinical tests and ultrasonography. After 6 months, radiographs: look for Von Rosen's line (45° abduction line is drawn through femoral shaft and should point to the acetabulum) and Perkins' line (femoral head epiphysis should lie below a horizontal line through the triradiate cartilage, medial to the vertical line drawn from the outer acetabular edge). Treatment: 3–6 months: double nappies for 6 weeks; 6 months: abduction splint. If still unstable, 6–18 months: traction, plaster spica or open surgery. If unsuccessful, 18 months–10 years: traction followed by surgery and 3 months of hip spica. Treatment after this time, or after 6 years in bilateral cases – should be avoided during development to prevent avascular necrosis of femoral head.

4. A **slipped upper femoral epiphysis** is a posterior displacement of the upper femoral epiphysis, usually in boys aged 14–16 years who are overweight or tall and thin. It is caused by a hormonal imbalance and trauma, producing a limp, pain and leg shortening.

5. **Protrusio acetabuli** is a pelvic deformity where the medial wall of the acetabulum expands inwards. It is associated with skeletal dysplasias, coxa vara, osteoarthritis, connective tissue disorders, Marfan syndrome, haemophilia and post-radiotherapy.

6. **Perthes' disease** is avascular necrosis of the femoral head occurring in boys (4:1, male:female) aged 4–10 years due to changing blood supply from the metaphysis to the epiphysis: this may be compromised by a joint effusion. Remodelling results in an abnormally shaped femoral head.

7. True shortening is due to joint or bony abnormality of the hip, knee or lower leg, and is determined by comparing the distances from the greater trochanter to the lateral malleolus on each side. Apparent shortening is seen when malalignment between the ankles (on lying) is caused by pelvic tilting, as occurs in a fixed adduction deformity. Measurement from the umbilicus or symphysis pubis highlights the difference between the sides.

8. **Osteoarthritis:** asymmetrical narrowing of the joint space with sclerosis of subcondylar bone, cysts close to the joint surface and osteophytes at the joint margin. **Rheumatoid arthritis:** periarticular osteoporosis,

marginal bony erosion, narrowing of joint space. At later stages, destruction and deformity, with subluxation of the joint surfaces.

9/10. **Analgesia:** paracetamol is preferred to long-term non-steroidal anti-inflammatory drugs. Physiotherapy and the use of a walking stick reduce weight bearing. With progressive pain and limitation in mobility and activity, surgery is considered. Initially a subtrochanteric osteotomy but, in late cases, an arthrodesis or a prosthetic joint replacement may be required.

11. **Early** (intra-operative) complications of total hip replacement include femoral shaft fracture and sciatic nerve damage (particularly with a posterior approach). **Intermediate** complications include deep venous thrombosis and pulmonary embolism; dislocation and infection. Chronic infection requires removal and delayed replacement of the prosthesis. **Late** complications include heterotopic bone formation causing pain and stiffness that may respond to anti-inflammatory medication. Other problems are aseptic loosening of the prosthesis and osteolysis, that may occur around the cement, polyethylene or metal particles.

12. Young patients, particularly those still undertaking active contact sports because any subsequent revision is accompanied by a much higher complication rate; mild disease; severe degenerative disease with destruction of the hip joint or multiple joint involvement; when there is doubt as to the origin of the hip pain such as with coexistent scoliotic problems; patient refusal or mental apathy towards the procedure; severe comorbidity; and obesity.

13. **Garden's classification:**
- I Incomplete impacted fracture
- II Complete undisplaced fracture
- III Moderately displaced fracture
- IV Severely displaced fracture.

   Grades I and II undisplaced can be managed with cannulated hip screws.

   Displacement disrupts the blood supply of bone, reducing the chances of natural healing and together with extra-capsular fractures are indication for radical surgery, extending to total hip replacement.

16 The knee

THE HISTORY

If you have a patient with a knee complaint in the long case, bring out the following aspects in your presentation.

Pain

- Ask the usual questions about pain (see page 25).
- Be very clear as to whether the pain is generalised or localised; the former suggests inflammatory or degenerative, the latter a mechanical cause.
- Tell the patient to point with one finger to where the pain is felt maximally.
- Ask if there is pain *above* the knee.
- Ask if it is exacerbated by walking or walking up and down stairs.

Stiffness

Ask if this is worse in the morning, on movement or after staying in one position, post-inactivity suggests arthritis.

Swelling

If preceded by an injury:

- Did the swelling occur straight away – suggesting a haemarthrosis?
- Did the swelling occur after a few hours?

Episodes of locking or giving way

Explain to the patient exactly what you mean by these terms. 'Locking' is the sudden inability to extend the knee fully. 'Giving way' describes the feeling of apprehension on weight bearing (see case 3 page 181).

THE EXAMINATION

As with the hip, examination of the knee will probably be relatively unfamiliar: practise on each other.

Don't worry too much about the 'additional assessment', eg the apprehension test and McMurray's test. Most of your examiners are not orthopaedic surgeons and just want to see that you have a basic routine of **LOOK, GAIT, FEEL, MEASURE, MOVE**.

Never forget to ask to see the patient *walk* at the end of the examination. This will also give you the opportunity of looking at the popliteal fossa for posterior knee swellings.

'Examine this patient's knee'

ACTION	NOTE
Introduce yourself	
Say what you wish to do	
Ask the patient's permission to proceed	
Expose both legs with the patient lying down	

ACTION	NOTE
STAND Ask patient to stand up Look from: • in front • the side • the back Ask patient to walk away from and then towards you	Genu valgum and varum are best seen in the standing position *?genu valgum/varum* *?genu recurvatum* *?swelling in popliteal fossa* gait: *?short-stepping* *?limp*

LOOK Compare the two sides	skin: *?erythema*
	             ?scars
	swelling: *?prepatellar*
	             ?infrapatellar
	             ?effusion
	             ?Bakers cyst

MEASURE Measure the circumference of each leg at a fixed point above the tibial tuberosity, eg 20 cm above and 15 cm below (document)	Initial quadriceps wasting can be detected just medial to the upper part of the patella
FEEL **a. Temperature** Run the back of your hand over both legs anteriorly and down each side	*?warm*
b. Tests for effusion *Bulge test* Empty the medial compartment by massaging up the medial side of the joint	Positive with very *little* fluid present

ACTION	NOTE
Retain fluid in the suprapatellar bursa with medial pressure from one hand	
Stroke down lateral side of the joint with your other hand, watching the medial side	*?appearance of ripple on flattened medial surface*
Patellar tap	Positive with *large* effusion
Empty the suprapatellar bursa: use your left hand to press downwards and backwards above the patella	
Keep this hand in position	
Push the patella sharply back with your right hand	*?feel/hear tap of patella on femur*
c. Palpation of joint line	The joint line is lower than you think
Bend the knee to about 90°	
Palpate the *medial* joint line: locate the tibial tuberosity and move your finger medially and proximally	tenderness: *?localised – joint line = meniscus; above and below joint line = colateral ligament*
	?generalised
	synovium: *?thickened*
	cartilage: *?swelling*
Palpate firmly, anterior to posterior	
Ask if/when it hurts	
Palpate the *lateral* joint line, moving your finger laterally and proximally from the tibial tuberosity	
Palpate the popliteal fossa	*?swelling*

ACTION	NOTE
MOVE (active, passive, resisted)	
Flexion and extension	
Ask patient to bend and then straighten his or her leg	range of active movement: *?limited flexion/extension*
Ask if/when it hurts	
Place your hand over the extended knee	
Try to flex and extend the knee joint yourself, left hand holding knee – and feeling for crepitus – right holding lower leg	range of passive movement: *?limited flexion/extension* *?crepitus*
Try to hyperextend the leg by lifting the heel upwards from the bed	*?hyperextension – normal 5–10°*
SPECIAL TESTS	
a. Ligament stability	
Medial collateral ligament	*?excess movement*
Place one hand on the *lateral* side of the *knee* and the other on the *medial* side of the ankle	compare both sides *?pain*
Try to push the ankle laterally while pushing the knee medially	
Lateral collateral ligament	*?excess movement*
Place one hand on the *medial* side of the *knee* and the other on the *lateral* side of the *ankle*	compare both sides *?pain*
Try to push the ankle medially while pushing the knee laterally	*?gap sign* (opening up of lateral joint line)
Anterior cruciate ligament	
Flex the knee to 90°	
Steady foot by sitting close (not on it)	
Palpate the hamstrings to ensure that they are relaxed	

ACTION	NOTE
Place thumbs of both your hands on the tibial tuberosity	*?tibia displaced anteriorly on femur* (positive anterior drawer sign)
Grasp the lower leg and pull it towards you	There may be a false-positive anterior drawer sign if the posterior cruciate ligament is ruptured
Posterior cruciate ligament Repeat above test but push the tibia *away* from you	*?tibia displaced posteriorly on femur* (positive posterior drawer sign)
b. The apprehension test Hold the patella laterally with the knee extended	Only perform this test if you suspect patellar instability
Bend the knee slowly	
Watch patient's face	*?resistance to further movement*
c. McMurray's test Flex the knee,	Only perform this test if, holding the joint steady, you suspect a torn meniscus
Use your other hand to rotate the foot slowly and fully extend the joint medially; repeat laterally	*?resistance to further movement* *?pain* *?click*
Examine the ankle pulses and sensation over the toes. Tell the examiner you would like to examine the joint above and below, and X-ray in two planes	
COMPLETE THE EXAMINATION Make sure that patient is comfortable	
Turn to the examiner	
Present your findings	

TYPICAL CASES

As with the hip, pain is the most common presenting symptom. It may be associated with stiffness and mechanical problems. The aetiology of knee pain in the aged is usually **arthritic**, while the contact activities of young adults make them subject to **mechanic problems**. There are also a large collection of other problems that give knee pain, including paediatric conditions and referred pain – these are first considered in Case 1. **NB** pain in the knee: always examine the hip.

1. KNEE PAIN

First ask yourself if the pain is due to knee pathology or if it is referred.

	Knee pathology	Referred pain
Localised?	Yes	No
Any pain above knee?	No	Yes
Exacerbated by walking?	Yes	Variable

Case 1: non-arthritic knee pain

The conditions comprise **congenital** and **acquired**, the latter being **traumatic** or **non-traumatic**. Traumatic may be **intra-capsular** (producing a haemarthrosis within an hour) or an **extra-capsular** injury. Non-traumatic conditions can classified by their position, and as common, paediatric and uncommon.

Anterior Knee Pain

a Patellofemoral and patellotendinopathy problems are common, frequently follow injury: they are characteristically exacerbated by:
- Going up and down stairs
- Sitting for a long time with the knee flexed
- Quadriceps wasting (particularly the lower fibres of vastus medialis)
- Small effusions, accentuated by activity

b In children consider:
- Osgood –Slatter's disease
- Growth spurt (especially adolescent girls)
- Chodromalacia patellae (especially adolescent boys)

- Osteochondritis dissecans
- Obesity
- Referred hip pain (NB an important differential)

c Uncommon - bursitis and fat pad impingement
Lateral Knee Pain
- Ilio-tibial band (ITB) friction syndrome
- Lateral collateral ligament damage
- OA knee

Medial Knee Pain
- Meniscal damage
- Medial collateral ligament damage
- Pes anserinus tendinopathy

Posterior Knee Pain
- Popliteal cysts
- Baker's cyst

Investigation: diagnosis can be made clinically but is confirmed radiologically; radiographs also demonstrate the extent of bone injury. MRI adds information on soft-tissue disease, while arthroscopy allows both diagnosis and treatment of intra-articular problems.

Treatment:
- Soft tissue injuries to the collateral ligaments are immobilised with a high knee brace followed by physiotherapy
- In cruciate ligament damage, as with hamstring conditions, physiotherapy and rehabilitation can negate the need for surgical reconstruction
- Meniscal injuries inevitably require arthroscopy and partial meniscectomy, but peripheral early tears may be sutured
- Patellofemoal disorders require biomechanical assessment and rigorous quadriceps physiotherapy
- Trauma with tibial plateau fractures inevitably require open reduction and fixation: with aspiration of the joint and elevation, progressing to cast brace for early mobilisation. Traction may also be applied when osteoporosis is present. Undisplaced patellar fractures can be managed with a backslab and mobilisation but displaced fractures may require wiring followed by a cast brace.
- In tuberculous disease, a full drug course must be given. Subsequent management may include that of osteoarthritic changes.
- Osteoarthritis and rheumatoid arthritis are treated as summarised in Case 2.

Case 2: arthritides

Compare and contrast the symptoms and signs of rheumatoid arthritis and osteoarthritis.

	Osteoarthritis	Rheumatoid arthritis
Pain	+ +	+ +
Stiffness	+	+ +
Palpable synovium	–	+ +
Deformity	Genu varum	Genu valgum
Effusion	+	+ +
Limitation of movement	+ +	+ +
Crepitus	+ +	+ +
Joint instability	–	+

Ask specifically about the *pattern* of stiffness: this may tell you about the joint pathology.

	Osteoarthritis	Rheumatoid arthritis
Morning stiffness	Sometimes	Very common
Time for morning stiffness to diminish	10–20 min (approx)	30 min–1 h (approx)
Stiffness after staying in one position	+ +	+

If you are asked to examine the knee in a short case, always glance at the hands. This will give you a clue if your patient has rheumatoid arthritis.

Remember: the knee may be the only joint involved in osteoarthritis; in rheumatoid arthritis, it is usually involved as part of a generalised syndrome (for hands see page 198).

Look carefully for scars of previous operations: your patient may have had a joint replacement. Look also at the thigh: note that in all knee injuries there is rapid muscle wasting of the thigh muscles, particularly of the medial quadriceps.

Treatment: osteoathritis of the knee is treated with analgesics and knee elastic support, progressing to depomedrone intra-articular injection and washout of degenerative material. If symptoms progress, other measures may include patellectomy, tibial osteotomy, prosthetic joint replacement or arthrodesis. Treatment of rheumatoid arthritis involves treating the generalised disease and, in the knee, arthroscopic synovectomy. When symptoms are not controlled by drugs, osteotomy is undertaken for marked valgus deformity and prosthetic joint replacement for extensive joint destruction. In both diseases, haemarthrosis and effusions are aspirated. Physiotherapy is an important aspect of rehabilitation.

Case 3: mechanical problems ('locking and giving way')

You would be extremely unlikely to have a patient with an acute injury in the examination, but there could be a patient with recurrent episodes.

True locking occurs with menisceal tears in plica syndrome (trapping of a synovial fold) and *loose bodies* ('joint mice'). Know the **causes of joint mice:**

- Osteochondritis dissecans

- Synovial chondromalacia

- Osteochondral fracture

- Localised separation of articular cartilage.

Pseudo locking is due to pain and apprehension. A knee **'gives way'** in patellofemoral disease and when there is any weakness of quadriceps, especially vastus medialis.

Treatment: when loose bodies or meniscal tears are present, arthroscopy allows diagnosis and treatment of the underlying problem, removing loose bodies and any damaged cartilage. If the anterior cruciate ligament requires replacement or repair for tears or knee instability, followed by a hinged knee brace and 12–18 months rehabilitation.

Case 4: knee deformities

You should know the causes of the two most common deformities: **genu valgum** and **genu varum**.

	Genu varum (bow legs)	Genu valgum (knock knees)
Physiological	Babies	Toddlers aged 3–4 (permissible to have 10 cm between ankles)
Arthritides	Osteoarthritis – cartilage loss in medial compartment	Rheumatoid arthritis
Metabolic	Vitamin C and D deficiency	Vitamin C and D deficiency
Growth disorders	• Paget's disease • Epiphyseal injury • Dysplasias, eg Blount's disease	• Epiphyseal injury • Dysplasias

Treatment: see Case 2.

2. KNEE SWELLINGS

Most lumps in and around the knee are due to bursitis or diverticula. Know the differential diagnosis.

a. Anterior (rare)

• Prepatellar bursa (housemaid's knee)

• Infrapatellar bursa (clergyman's knee)

• Osgood–Schlatter disease.

b. Lateral/medial (rare)

• Cyst of lateral meniscus

• Cyst of medial meniscus

- Exostosis.

c. Posterior

- Semimembranous bursa

- Baker's cyst

- Popliteal aneurysm.

You should be able to recognise a bursa by the following features:

- Not tender (unless infected)

- Smooth surface

- Fluctuant

- Transilluminable

- May be attached to skin

- Immobile.

Case 5: anterior knee swellings

a. Prepatellar bursitis: housemaid's knee

Here the swelling is *over* the patella. Ask the patient his or her occupation: it is common in carpet layers, tilers and roofers, but not so common in housewives!

b. Infrapatellar bursitis: clergyman's knee

Here the swelling is distal to the patella.

c. Osgood–Schlatter disease

Suspect this condition in an adolescent who complains of pain after physical activity: look for a lump over the tibial tuberosity. On palpation, it is usually tender.

Treatment: bursae and cysts are usually managed conservatively but may, if infected, need aspiration and appropriate antibiotics.

Case 6: posterior knee swellings

a. Semimembranous bursitis

The swelling is behind the knee in the medial part of the popliteal fossa, above the joint line.

b. Baker's cyst/popliteal cyst

This is a synovial diverticulum extending into the popliteal fossa through a deficit in the posterior capsule. The swelling is behind the knee, below the joint line. You may be asked to distinguish the terms 'popliteal cyst' and 'Baker's cyst':

Popliteal cyst:

- No underlying pathology

- Seen in young adults/children.

Baker's cyst:

- Pathology of rest of knee, eg rheumatoid arthritis, osteoarthritis, gout, tuberculosis

- Often exacerbates pre-existing symptoms, eg further interference with knee flexion.

c. Popliteal aneurysm

This is easily detected because of its expansile pulsation:

- Always palpate the other leg (it may be bilateral)

- Examine the peripheral pulses

- Palpate the abdomen and groin for associated aortic and femoral aneurysms.

Treatment: bursae and cysts (see Case 5). Popliteal aneurysms require surgical repair to prevent acute ischaemia from thrombosis or rupture.

Case 7: Knee injuries

Remember that the knee contains not only the femorotibial joint, but also a joint between the patella and the femur. Always check for fractures along the entire length of the fibula.

Knee injuries can cause:

a. Bone fractures:

- Tibial plateau fractures occur as a result of the femur compressing the tibia.

- Supracondylar femoral fractures may damage the popliteal artery.

- Fractures of the patella may be transverse (split in half) or comminuted (shattered). Patellar fractures, quadriceps tendon tears or tears of the patellar ligament can all give rise to loss of the extensor mechanism of the knee.

b. Ligamentous injury: sudden change of direction of movement exerted on the knee can cause anterior cruciate ligament (ACL) injury. This can be associated with a positive anterior drawer test (anterior translation of the tibia on the femur when knee is flexed at 90°, meniscial damage and haemarthrosis (blood in the knee joint). Severe trauma can give rise to the Terrible Triad of O'Donohue (anterial cruciate, medial meniscus, medial collateral ligament damage).

c. Joint dislocation:

- Patellar dislocation occurs laterally. It may reduce spontaneously on extension of the knee.

- Knee dislocation is relatively rare and requires high-velocity trauma; it may give rise to injuries to the popliteal artery and the peroneal nerve, as well as to major ligamentous injuries. This is unlikely in this case.

- In such cases also consider damage to the joints above and below, eg impacted fracture of the neck of femur and ankle sprains. **Remember:** pain in knee – examine the hip.

FAQS AND POPULAR VIVA QUESTIONS

1. What is the normal angle of the femur on the tibia?

2. What are the causes of genu varum?

3. What are the causes of genu valgum?

4. What is the cause of Osgood–Schlatter disease?

5. What is osteochondritis dissecans?

6. What are the causes of anterior knee pain?

7. What are the causes of a 'locked knee'?

8. What radiological features would you see in osteoarthritis?

9. What radiological features would you see in rheumatoid arthritis?

10. Where is the most common site for a meniscus to tear? How would such an injury present?

ANSWERS

1. The tibiofemoral angle is 5–7° of femoral valgus. It is usually greater in the female due to the wider pelvis.

2. **Genu varum** (bow legs): >6 cm between the knees when the heels are together. Physiological normal finding in babies; abnormal growth of the posteromedial proximal tibial epiphysis; osteoarthritis and cartilage loss in the medial compartment; Paget's disease and epiphyseal injury; vitamin C and D deficiency.

3. Genu valgum: >8 cm between malleoli with knees touching. Physiological normal variant in toddlers aged 3–4; rheumatoid arthritis; dysplasias; epiphyseal injury; vitamin C and D deficiency.

4. Painful swelling of the **tibial tubercle** in adolescence due to traction injury of the apophysis. Spontaneous recovery with alteration of activity.

5. **Avascular necrosis** of subchondral bone: avascular fragments separate and may give rise to loose bodies.

6. **Congenital lesions** (eg bipartite patella); injuries; stress; (growth spurts, chondromalacia patellae, obesity, plica syndrome); osteochondritis (Osgood–Schlatter disease, osteochondritis dissecans); bursae (bursitis); joint pathology (rheumatoid arthritis, osteoarthritis, tuberculosis).

7. **Meniscal tear** (including bucket handle); loose bodies (joint mice) such as in osteochondritis dissecans; synovial chondromalacia; osteochondral fracture; localised separation of articular cartilage and plica syndrome (trapping of a synovial fold).

8. **Osteoarthritis:** asymmetrical narrowing of joint space, sclerosis of subcondylar bone; cysts close to the joint surface and osteophytes at the joint margin.

9. **Rheumatoid arthritis:** periarticular osteoporosis, marginal bony erosion, narrowing of joint space. At later stages, destruction and deformity, with subluxation of joint surfaces.

10. Splitting is usually along the length of the **medial meniscus:** bucket-handle tears remain attached at each end. It presents with severe pain, usually on the medial side of the knee, often as a sports injury. The knee is typically locked in flexion. Swelling follows a few hours or days later. Recurrent and chronic problems may requir surgery.

17 The hand and foot

THE HISTORY

Hand and foot problems usually come up as short cases and OSCEs. You may be told to ask the patient a few questions: first ask about the patient's main complaint. Then go through the usual questions about pain and swelling (page 25 and 40), and autoimmune conditions.

Ask specifically about loss of function and social history:

- Can you hold a cup and feed yourself easily?

- Can you turn a doorknob?

- Do you have difficulty dressing yourself, eg doing up buttons?

- Are you right or left handed

- Do you have difficulty washing yourself?

- Can you write?

- What job do you do?

THE EXAMINATION

The instruction will usually be to 'examine this person's hands'. Seek clues as to the underlying cause right from the beginning.

Look at both sides:

- Elbows: *?rheumatoid nodules*

- Nails and skin: *?nail, ?pitting, ?psoriasis (and scalp) ?scarring of systemic sclerosis (and face)*

- Ears: *?gouty tophi.*

'Examine this patient's hand(s)'

ACTION	NOTE
Introduce yourself	
Say what you wish to do	
Ask the patient's permission to proceed	
Place a pillow on the patient's lap and tell the patient to rest *both* hands on it	

LOOK

Observe:

Dorsal surface	skin:	*?thin/bruised*
		?tattoos
		?purpura
		?spider naevi
	nails:	*?clubbing/pitting/ pallor/cyanosis*
	muscle:	*?wasting of dorsal interossei*
	joints:	*?swelling* (Heberden's or Bouchard's nodes)
	bony deformities:	
		?rheumatoid arthritis (page 198)
Palmar surface	skin:	*?erythema*
		?Dupuytren's contracture
	muscles:	
		?wasting of thenar/hypothenar eminence and palmar interossei
From the side (patient's hands outstretched)		*?finger drop*
		?break in normal finger cascade

ACTION	NOTE
Knuckles (patient's fists clenched)	*?swelling of MCP joints*
Hands in praying position	Examine bulk of thenar and back-to-back hypothenar eminences: *?same on both sides*
FEEL	
Ask if the hands are painful	
Run the back of your hand over the patient's forearm and fingers	
Compare the temperature of both sides	*?warm/warmer/moist*
Palpate and squeeze gently over:	
• MCP joints 2–5	
• IP joints 2–5	*?soft tissue swelling*
	?bony swelling
	?areas of maximum tenderness
Palpate and squeeze gently over:	
• thumb joints	*?soft tissue swelling*
• radiocarpal joint	*?bony swelling*
• inferior radioulnar joint	*?areas of maximum tenderness*
MOVE	
Place your thumb on the patient's palm and move each MCP and IP joint in turn	*?limited range of movement* *?crepitus from flexor tendon*
TEST POWER	
Ask patient to grip two of your fingers as hard as possible	*?strength of power grip*
Ask patient to oppose thumb to index finger as hard as possible	

ACTION	NOTE
Hook your index finger under point of contact	
Try to pull it through	*?strength of precision grip*
Test thumb abduction: 'Point your thumb up towards your nose. Now keep it there and don't let me push it downwards'	*?strength of abductor pollicis longus* (median nerve)
Test finger abduction: 'Spread your fingers wide apart. Don't let me push them together'	*?strength of interossei* (ulnar nerve)
Test finger adduction: 'Grip this sheet of paper between two fingers at a time'	*?strength of interossei* (ulnar nerve)

TEST SENSATION

Compare sensation on each side gently with a sterile needle over:

• index finger	median nerve
• little finger	ulnar nerve
• lateral aspect of thumb base	radial nerve

ASSESS FUNCTION

Ask patient to undo a button	
Ask patient to write his or her name	

ASSESS FURTHER	Perform the following tests only if appropriate

If you suspect ulnar nerve lesion:

Froment's sign

Ask patient to grasp a piece of paper between the thumb and index finger (using both hands). Try to pull paper away	*?flexing of terminal phalanx as you pull away* (flexor pollicis brevis compensating for weak adductor pollicis brevis–ulnar nerve)

ACTION	NOTE
If you suspect carpal tunnel syndrome:	
a. Tinel's sign	
Percuss over the distal skin crease of wrist	*?pain/tingling felt over lateral palm*
b. Phalen's test	
Hold the patient's wrist maximally flexed for 1 min	*?pain/tingling felt over lateral palm*
If patient cannot flex an IP joint:	
Hold middle phalanx still	*?flexion present* (indicates flexor digitorum profundus intact)
Flex distal phalanx	
Hold all fingers in extension except the one to be tested	
Tell patient to flex that finger	*?flexion present* (indicates flexor digitorum superficialis intact)
If you suspect de Quervain's tenosynovitis:	
Finkelstein's test	
Ask patient to grasp his or her thumb in the adjacent palm	*?pain* (indicates de Quervain's tenosynovitis)
Now deviate the fist towards the ulnar side	

If you are asked to examine a patient's foot, follow the usual routine of 'LOOK, FEEL, MOVE, MEASURE', examining each joint in turn as outlined on page 154. There will usually be an obvious abnormality which you should describe systematically before giving your diagnosis.

TYPICAL CASES

1. THE HAND

Case 1: contracted hand

You may be shown a contracted hand. Your differential diagnosis will include an **ulnar nerve palsy** (page 195) and **Klumpke's palsy** (page 196) which both result in a clawed hand. A contracted hand can result from the following conditions.

	Cause	Joints affected
Dupuytren's contracture	• Autosomal dominant inheritance • Alcohol/cirrhosis • Phenytoin • Diabetes mellitus • AIDS, tuberculosis	*Flexion* of MCP and PIP joints (affects ring and little fingers)
Volkmann's contracture	Trauma at/below elbow leads to ischaemia of forearm muscles	*Flexion* of MCP and IP joints. Can be straightened only when wrist is flexed
Shortening of intrinsic hand muscles	• Spasticity • Scarring due to trauma/infection	*Flexion* of MCP joints *Extension* of IP joints *Adduction* of thumb Bunnel's test: active and passive IP flexion limited when MCP joint held in extension as well as flexed

The most common cause of a contracted hand is **Dupuytren's contracture:**

- Feel for the hard, subcutaneous nodules on the palmar surface – usually involving the 4th and 5th digits.

- Look at the knuckles, which may also be thickened (Garrod's pads).

- Look at the other hand.

- Ask to examine the soles of the feet: similar nodules may be felt.

If permitted, ask the following questions to determine the cause:

- Do you drink alcohol? How much per day? Do you have any liver problems?

- Do you have diabetes?

- Do you suffer from epilepsy? Are you on phenytoin?

Treatment: Dupuytren's contracure is usually managed conservatively but where there is progressive flexion of ring and middle fingers the patient is unable to have a flat palm when placed on a table.
The thickened fascia may be excised (faciectomy or dermofaciectomy graft; if skin involved) with splintage for 6–12 weeks postoperatively. In severe, persisting, disabling deformity the little finger may have to be amputated.

Volkmann's contracture and shortening of the intrinsic hand muscles are usually managed conservatively although muscle release procedures and tendon transfers may be possible.

Case 2: median nerve lesion

This is usually **carpal tunnel syndrome**. You may be asked the associations. Classify your answer:

- Endocrine causes (acromegaly, myxoedema)

- Connective tissue diseases (rheumatoid arthritis)

- Fluid retention (congestive cardiac failure, pregnancy)

- Trauma.

Remember the signs:

a. Sensory loss: over lateral three and a half digits.

Note that the palm may be spared as the palmar branch of the median nerve passes superficial to the flexor retinaculum.

b. Motor loss and wasting, affects **LOAF**:

Lumbricals (lateral two)

Opponens pollicis

Abductor pollicis brevis (easiest to detect)

Flexor pollicis brevis

c. *Positive Tinel's sign and Phalen's test* (see examination scheme, page 192).

Treatment: see after Case 6.

Case 3: ulnar nerve palsy

This is usually due to trauma at the elbow: look for scars here. It may occasionally arise from repeated trauma to the heel of the hand, in which case there is no sensory loss. Revise the signs:

a. Position: claw hand.

b. Sensory loss: over little and ring fingers.

c. Motor loss and wasting: affects the interossei; most noticeable dorsally. There is weakened finger abduction and adduction.

d. Positive Froment's sign (see page 191).

Treatment: see after Case 6.

Case 4: radial nerve palsy

The most common cause is when the patient falls asleep with his or her arm hanging over the edge of the chair ('Saturday night palsy'). Remember that the radial nerve lies in the spiral groove and can therefore also be damaged by fractures of the shaft of the humerus.

The main signs are wrist drop and wasting of the posterior forearm muscles. There is very little sensory loss – only over the anatomical snuffbox.

Treatment: see after Case 6.

Case 5: Erb's palsy (C5, C6 roots)

The most common causes are birth trauma and injury. The signs are as follows:

a. Position: arm internally rotated with the forearm pronated and the palm facing backwards (the waiter's tip sign).

b. Sensory loss: over deltoid.

c. Muscle weakness and wasting: affects deltoid, most of shoulder rotator muscles, biceps and brachioradialis.

d. Reflexes: absent biceps and supinator reflexes.

Treatment: see after Case 6.

Case 6: Klumpke's palsy (T1 root)

This can be caused by a cervical rib or apical lung tumour (Pancoast's tumour): remember to check for an associated **Horner syndrome** – miosis, ptosis, enophthalmos and anhidrosis of the face.

The hand is clawed and wasted. There is sensory loss over the inner aspect of the arm and forearm.

Treatment: where the nerve injury is neuropraxia, there may be some spontaneous recovery. For more severe injuries, the site of damage must be identified and immediate repair may be possible. Recovery is more likely in children and in pure motor or sensory nerves. Brachial plexus injuries involving avulsion of the nerve roots are not amenable to surgery and a useless, flail, upper limb is an occasional indication for amputation. Progress of healing can be followed by a positive Tinel's sign.

Case 7: dropped finger

Usually affects little and ring fingers. Finger can be passively extended but drops down upon release.

Cause: extensor tendon rupture (close to ulnar styloid and rheumatoid arthritis).

Treatment: tendon repair.

Case 8: mallet finger

Terminal IP joint cannot be extended.

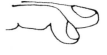

Cause: division/avulsion of extensor digitorum longus (at base of distal phalanx).

Treatment: a splint in the acute phase, retaining hyperextension of the distal interphalangeal joint. Old injuries with marked deformity may require tendon reconstruction

Case 9: boutonnière deformity

- Flexion of PIP joint

- Hyperextension of DIP joint.

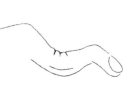

Cause: rupture of central slip of extensor expansion. Associated with rheumatoid arthritis and trauma.

Treatment: surgical correction, by transferring the lateral slip of the tendon to the middle phalanx.

Case 10: swan-neck deformity
(opposite of boutonnière deformity)

- Hyperextension of PIP joint

- Flexion of DIP joint

Cause: associated with rheumatoid arthritis.

Treatment: painful deformed and defective hands might be relieved by synovectomy, with or without prosthetic replacement of the MCP and IP joints.

Case 11: trigger finger/stenosing tenosynovitis

- Patient's finger clicks when it is bent

- When patient straightens out hand, affected finger remains bent and then straightens with a click

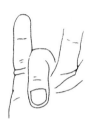

- Feel for a tender nodule over the tendon sheath, over the distal palmar crease.

Cause: inflammatory thickening of the tendon or its sheath.

Treatment: steroid injection; if fails, the stenotic area of the tendon sheath is incised to release and allow free movement of the tendon.

Case 12: rheumatoid arthritis

This is a very common short case. You should be able to describe the characteristic deformities:

- Ulnar deviation of the fingers

- Boutonnière deformity

- Swan-neck deformity

- Z-deformity of the thumb

- Subluxation of the MCP joints

- Dorsal subluxation of the ulna at the carpal joint (piano key sign).

Also look for additional features:

- Swelling of the PIP joints

- Wasting of the small hand muscles

- Atrophic skin and purpura (secondary to steroid therapy).

Palpate the elbows for rheumatoid nodules.

Treatment: painful, deformed and defective hands might be helped by synovectomy, with or without prosthetic replacement of the MCP and IP joints.

Case 13: osteoarthritis

Note especially:

- Heberden's nodes: bony thickening of DIP joints
- Bouchard's nodes: bony thickening of the PIP joints
- Squaring of thumb: involvement of carpometacarpal joint of thumb.

Treatment is usually conservative:

- Simple analgesia
- Discontinue any activity likely to aggravate wear and tear of cartilage
- Splints and physiotherapy
- More rarely, steroid injection or surgical therapy.

Case 14: the wasted hand

This is a common short case. The two most common causes of generalised hand wasting are old age and rheumatoid arthritis. However, remember neurological causes:

- Palpate for a cervical rib.
- Look for scars around the elbow (ulnar nerve palsy).
- Test abductor pollicis brevis and the interossei for median and ulnar nerve palsies respectively.

Treatment: if a T1 nerve injury is identified, the offending cervical rib or compressing band must be removed or released surgically as soon as possible.

Case 15: fall on an outstretched hand (FOOSH)

Falls in the elderly are a major cause of morbidity due to osteoporosis which increases the risk of fracture, as well as poor mobility, balance and vision, which make falling more likely.

Fractures can occur in the carpal bones of the wrist, the radius or ulna, as well as in more proximal joints such as the shoulder due to pressure transmission.

You must consider three injuries:

1. **Colles' fracture:** fracture of the distal end of the radius bone, with shortening, and dorsal diplacement and angulation of the fractured distal segment. This gives the classic 'dinner-fork' deformity of the wrist and is typical of a fall on an outstretched hand. The wrist can be 'pulled' (reduced) using local anaesthesia (into haematoma or a biers block), sedation and analgesia; or it can be manipulated under anaesthesia, followed by fixation in a plaster cast. Complex fractures may require open reduction and internal fixation (ORIF). Persistent deformity and poor wrist function are common complications of inadequate reduction and immobilisation.

2. **Smith's fracture:** fracture of the distal radius with volar angulation (opposite to Colles') of the fractured segment. This occurs when the impact occurs on the dorsum of the hand.

3. **Scaphoid fracture (more common at a younger age):** the patient is tender over the anatomical snuffbox (space between the extensor tendons of the thumb: extensor policis longus vs extensor policis brevis and abductor policis longus). The pain can be reproduced by a telescoping movement of the thumb (as if trying to pull thumb out or push it in). Avascular necrosis of the proximal scaphoid segment can occur due to disturbance of the blood supply to it. Treatment normally involves immobilisation with a plaster from the upper forearm to just proximal to the metacarpophalangeal joints of the fingers, but including the metacarphphalyngeal joint of the thumb, with the wrist slightly extended (the glass holding position), for 6-8 weeks.

Case 16: shoulder injuries

Injuries to the shoulder can involve:

- Bones: fractures of the humerus, clavicle and scapula

- Joints: dislocation of joints between any of the above bones

- Muscles and ligaments: rotator cuff injuries.

1. **Humeral shaft fractures** may damage the brachial artery (anteriorly) and radial nerve (posteriorly). Clinical and radiological diagnosis are needed. Radial nerve damage presents with loss of wrist extension (motor) and loss of sensation over first dorsal web space of the hand (sensory).

2. **Shoulder dislocation:** over 90% of traumatic shoulder dislocations cause the humerus to lie anteriorly (anterior dislocations). The patient supports the dislocated humerus, while the shoulder contour is lost. Dislocations can cause axillary nerve and artery damage, with loss of sensation over the outer aspect of the upper arm (sergeant's patch / regimental patch area). Shoulder dislocations can be reduced using Kocher's method. Recurrent dislocation of the joint can occur.

3. **Clavicular fracture:** the clavicle commonly fractures in its middle third segment. The outer third becomes depressed by the weight of the arm, while the proximal third is elevated by the sternocleidomastoid muscle. The fractured clavicle is treated with an arm sling. Dimpling of skin over the fracture / proximity of bony spicules to skin mandates surgical intervention, as does significant displacement (the latter may damage the subclavian vessels or brachial plexus).

4. **Rotator cuff injuries:** may involve any of the short articular muscles, causing painful movements (rotar cuff; tendinitis). The supraspinatus may impinge on the acromion producing a painful arc on abduction. Transection of supraspinatus may be accompanied by an inability to initiate shoulder abduction. Treatment includes repair of torn rotator tendons and removal of any bony irregularities on the acromion.

2. THE FOOT

The three common foot problems you will see in an examination are hallux valgus, hammer toe and claw toes.

Case 17: hallux valgus (bunions)

This is lateral deviation of the great toe (valgus deformity) with protrusion of the metatarsal head. The condition is usually bilateral: always look at the other foot. Examine for the following features:

- Inflammation: heat and redness over the bunion
- Associated hammer toes, due to overlapping (crowding)
- Corns and callosities over and under the metatarsal heads
- Secondary osteoarthritis of the metatarsophalangeal joint.

Treatment: appropriate footwear (low heels, wide toes); surgical corrective osteotomy or arthrodesis.

Case 18: hammer toe

This usually affects the second toe. It can be bilateral. There is a fixed flexion deformity of the PIP joint.

Treatment: see Case 17.

Case 19: claw toes

Claw toes (hyperextension metatarsophalangeal, flexion interphalangeal joints): usually idiopathic. However, you should know the secondary causes:

- Rheumatoid arthritis
- Neurological problems, eg polio, Charcot–Marie–Tooth disease, diabetes.

Look for an associated pes cavus (high foot arch).

Treatment: these deformities are usually managed conservatively with appropriate footwear but the affected joints can be arthrodesed.

FAQS AND POPULAR VIVA QUESTIONS

THE HAND

1. What muscles do the median, ulnar and radial nerves supply in the hand?

2. What are the signs of median, ulnar and radial nerve palsies?

3. What are the causes of median, ulnar and radial nerve palsies?

4. In what position would you fix the hand after injury to avoid stiffness?

5. What is de Quervain's tenosynovitis?

6. What is a trigger finger?

7. What associations of Dupuytren's contracture do you know?

THE FOOT

8. Describe the deformity of club foot.

9. Are there any indications for treating flat feet?

10. What is hallux valgus? How would you manage it?

11. What is the difference between hallux valgus and hallux rigidus?

12. What are the causes of pes cavus and claw toes?

ANSWERS

1. **Median:** thenar muscles and lateral two lumbricals, flexor digitorum superficialis and lateral two tendons of flexor digitorum profundus. **Ulnar:** hypothenar muscles, adductor pollicis, tendons of flexor digitorum profundus to ring and little finger. **Radial:** posterior compartment muscles (the long extensor tendons are supplied by its posterior interosseous branch).

2. **Median:** thenar wasting, loss of thumb abduction, flexion of ulnar fingers but pointing of the index finger, loss of wrist flexion and pronation. Loss of sensation over the radial three and a half digits including the nail beds. **Ulnar:** loss of intrinsic muscle function of the hand produces a claw hand with loss of finger abduction and thumb adduction. Loss of sensation over the ulnar one and a half digits including the nail bed. Positive Froment's sign. **Radial:** loss of elbow extension with injuries to the upper arm; loss of extensors of wrist, fingers and thumb, and thumb abduction. Sensory loss over anatomical snuffbox.

3. **Median:** penetrating injuries in the arm and forearm, elbow dislocation, carpal dislocation, carpal tunnel syndrome due to fluid retention in association with congestive cardiac failure, pregnancy, connective tissue disease (rheumatoid arthritis), endocrine disease (acromegaly, myxoedema).

   Ulnar: usually disease around the elbow, eg fractures, dislocations, entrapment in the cubital tunnel syndrome, particularly with severe valgus deformity and osteoarthritis, compression injuries against the medial epicondyle (during anaesthesia or trauma), penetrating injuries in the forearm, repeated trauma over the pisohamate tunnel (in cyclists).

   Radial: falling asleep with the arm hanging over the back of a chair (Saturday night palsy), midshaft fracture of the humerus with damage in the spiral groove, penetrating injuries and fracture dislocation of the elbow.

   Prolonged use of a tourniquet or acute ischaemia can damage all three nerves.

4. Intrinsic plus position: wrist 10° extension; metacarpophalangeal 80° flexion; interphalangeal 0° – keeps collateral ligaments taught, preventing intrinsic shortening.

5. **De Quervain's tenosynovitis** is thickening, inflammation and tenderness of the tendon sheaths of extensor pollicis brevis and longus, and abductor pollicis longus, giving pain on thumb abduction against resistance and passive adduction.

6. Patient's finger clicks when it is bent and usually has to be forcibly straightened. A palpable tendon nodule over the distal palmar crease, may be present. Symptoms are due to trapping of the nodule by a stenosis in the sheath.

7. **Dupuytren's contracture** has an autosomal dominant inheritance, and is associated with alcoholic cirrhosis, phenytoin, diabetes mellitus, AIDS and tuberculosis.

8. In **club foot**, the ankle is in equines, the heel inverted and the forefoot adducted and supinated, so that the foot sole faces posteromedially. The foot cannot be dorsiflexed to touch the leg as is normal in neonates.

9. **Flat feet** are common and no treatments are required in asymptomatic children or adults. Treatment is indicated in tarsal conditions (fixed/fused tarsals) and failure of correction of the medial arch when on tiptoe. Initially plaster with foot in plantar grade position, if failure, surgical intervention.

10. In **hallux valgus**, there is excessive lateral angulation of the big toe away from the axis of the metatarsal. It can be treated by appropriate footwear and, when symptomatic (eg an infected bunion), the prominent part of the metatarsal head can be excised with a corrective osteotomy. Alternative surgical treatments include excision of the metatarsophalangeal joint or arthrodesis.

11. **Hallux rigidus** is stiffness of the first metatarsophalangeal joint. Causes include osteoarthritis, trauma, osteochondritis or gout, usually without the associated lateral angulation of the toe of hallux valgus.

12. **Pes cavus** is usually idiopathic but may be secondary to neurological disorders such as peroneal muscular atrophy or Friedreich's ataxia. It is often associated with clawing of the toes and with callosities under the metatarsal heads. The metatarsophalangeal joints are extended and the interphalangeal joints are flexed.

18 Arterial insufficiency of the lower limb

THE HISTORY

'Arteriopath' patients are readily available for examinations because of their age and complications. They are usually given as long cases, because the histories tend to be extensive. In your 'history of presenting complaint', include not only the symptoms of peripheral vascular disease, but also all other symptoms, risk factors, past history, and family history of cardiovascular and cerebrovascular and lower limb arterial disease.

Presenting symptoms

- Can you describe the pain in your legs? (Ask pain questions, see page 25)

- Does the pain come on when you walk/exercise?

- How far can you walk before you get the pain? (Claudication distance is best described in terms of a *known* distance, eg from the entrance of the hospital to the clinic.)

- When you stop walking, how long does it take for the pain to go away?

- Can you walk *through* the pain?

- How long have you had the problem? Has it got any better or worse over this time?

- How does it affect your lifestyle and does it interfere with your work?

- Have you any pain in your leg or foot at rest?

- What relieves your pain? (Rest pain may be relieved by walking about and hanging the leg over the side of the bed).

- Where is the pain in your leg (calf, thigh, buttock)?

In a man, ask about erectile function (Leriche syndrome).

Past surgical history

Ask about past surgery and investigations (duplex scans, angiograms) for peripheral vascular disease. When you present your history, describe these events chronologically and as concisely as possible.

Past medical history

Ask about previous myocardial infarcts/strokes/transient ischaemic attacks/leg ulcers.

Drugs and allergies

Ask about any known allergies to drugs.

Associated cardiovascular and cerebrovascular problems

Ask about chest pain/shortness of breath on exertion/palpitations/ankle swelling/loss of sensation or power of a limb/loss of vision/speech problems.

Risk factors

Ask about smoking /hypertension/diabetes/cholesterol levels.

Family history

Ask about a family history of cardiovascular/cerebrovascular/peripheral vascular disease.

Tailor the rest of your history towards the differential diagnosis – it is important to ask about neurological symptoms, such as paraesthesia in the leg, because there may be a neurological cause of the pain.

THE EXAMINATION

The OSLER/long case

Pay particular attention to the following:

- Peripheral vascular system: look for ulcers on pressure areas and over the tips and between the toes. Record all pulses and bruits on a diagram (see page 210); felt against underlying bone – ?enlarged

- Pulse: rate, rhythm, volume, vessel wall

- Heart

- Fundoscopy

- Neurological examination of the lower limb: in a patient complaining of leg pain, you may be asked to explain how your examination findings point to a diagnosis of claudication/rest pain rather than nerve root pain.

The OSCE/short case

Listen carefully to or read the instruction: if your examiner asks you to examine the patient's lower limb, do not jump straight into the following scheme, but follow the systematic approach outlined on page 151. Similarly, if asked to examine an ulcer on a limb, proceed as for the examination of any ulcer (pages 44–45).

'Examine this patient's lower limb peripheral vascular system'

ACTION	NOTE
Introduce yourself	
Say what you wish to do	
Ask the patient's permission to proceed	
Expose both legs completely	

ACTION	NOTE
LOOK	
Stand at the end of the bed and observe	colour: *?white/blue/black*
	trophic changes:
	?shiny skin
	?hair loss
	?loss of subcutaneous tissue
	?ulcers
Look at pressure points:	ulcers (pages 53–56):
• lateral side of foot	*?size*
• head of first metatarsal	*?shape/dimensions*
	?depth
• heel	*?edge*
• malleoli	*?base*
Observe:	
• tips of toes	metatarsal head: *diabetes*
• between toes	toes: *critical limb ischaemia*
	heel: *critical pressure ulcer*
	gaiter region: *venous ulceration*
FEEL	
Run the back of your hand along both limbs	*?warm/cold*
	?point of temperature change
Compare the two sides	
Press the tip of a toenail for 2 seconds	*?capillary refilling time*
Count the number of seconds for the nail to become pink again	

ACTION	NOTE
Feel pulses:	Compare right with left In the OSLER/long case; use a diagram to record pulses and bruits:

a. Femoral pulse: feel midway between symphysis pubis and ASIS (midinguinal point)

b. Popliteal pulse: ask the patient to bend his or her knee. Put your thumbs on the tibial tuberosity and feel pulse with eight fingertips

c. Dorsalis pedis: feel along cleft between first two metatarsals, lateral to extensor hallucis longus tendon. Use three fingers

?enlargement

ACTION	NOTE
d. Posterior tibial: halfway along line between medial malleolus and the prominence of the heel	
LISTEN	
Listen for bruits at all sites, ie along aorta, iliac, femoral and popliteal arteries, and over the adductor hiatus, on both sides	
ASSESS FURTHER	
Elevate leg about 15°	*?venous guttering*
Look	
Elevate leg further	*?angle at which leg becomes pale (Buerger's angle)*
Then ask patient to hang leg over side of bed (Buerger's test)	*?time of venous filling* *?reactive hyperaemia on dependency*
SAY	
'I would like to examine:	
• the rest of the peripheral vascular system	
• the heart	
• the abdomen for an aortic aneurysm'	
If asked to assess the rest of peripheral vascular system,	
Feel:	
• radial pulse	
• carotid pulse	

ACTION	NOTE
Listen for: • carotid bruit (just behind angle of mandible) • subclavian bruit (above middle of clavicle) • radiofemoral delay	

COMPLETE THE EXAMINATION

Make sure that your patient is comfortable

Cover the legs

Turn to your examiner and present your findings

TYPICAL CASES

It is extremely unlikely that you will have a patient with an acutely ischaemic limb in the examination because this is a surgical emergency. However, be aware of the causes of **acute ischaemia** and the symptoms and signs – remember the **6 P**s:

1. **P**ain

2. **P**araesthesia

3. **P**aralysis

4. **P**allor

5. **P**ulselessness

6. **P**erishingly cold.

Case 1: intermittent claudication

Don't worry if your history doesn't fit into any neat category: just report clearly and confidently on your findings. Ask yourself the following questions – this will help enormously in your presentation and discussion of the case with the examiners.

a. Is your patient's pain due to vascular disease?

It is quite possible that your patient has symptomless arterial disease with loss of pulses, but is suffering from a different cause of leg pain. Know the features of claudication pain:

- Cramp like

- Felt in the muscle

- Comes on invariably and only with exercise

- Stops after about 2 minutes of rest.

b. What is the differential diagnosis?

Think of the following:

Sciatica

This is differentiated from claudication by the following features:

- History of disc lesion/back trouble

- Pain felt in back, down buttock and thigh

- No characteristic relationship to exercise

- Limited straight-leg raising

- Neurological signs, eg wasting, loss of power, reflexes and sensation.

Osteoarthritis of the hip

This can be difficult to distinguish because the pain is also worsened by exercise. The pain is felt in the hip joint but can be referred to the knee. It varies from day to day.

Anterior tibial compartment syndrome (rare in an examination)

This occurs in young people after unaccustomed exercise. The pain is felt in the anterior part of the lower leg.

Cauda equina claudication

This is the most difficult to distinguish. There are two pathologies. Both lead to sciatic-like pain and to limited straight-leg raising after exercise:

- Disc pathology: partial compression of cauda equina by prolapsed disc

- Aortoiliac disease: on exercise, a drop in pressure leads to ischaemia of cauda equina.

c. What is the site of the main occlusion?

Try to relate your patient's symptoms (site of pain) and signs (absence of pulses, presence of bruits) to the anatomy. Early claudication – superficial femoral; thigh – common femoral; external iliac/profunda origin – unilateral buttock; bilateral buttock – aorta. A mental picture of the angiogram helps.

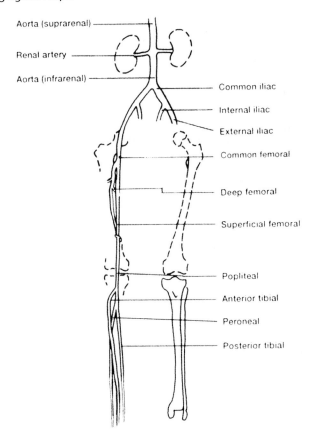

Distinguish between femorodistal disease and aortoiliac disease:

	Femorodistal disease	Aortoiliac disease
Site of pain	• Calf	• Calf • Thigh • Buttock
Absent pulses	• Foot • Popliteal	• Foot • Popliteal • Femoral

If aortoiliac symptoms are unilateral, occlusion is probably of the common iliac artery. If symptoms are bilateral (rare), occlusion may be of the aorta. Think of the tetrad of Leriche syndrome:

• Bilateral pain

• Impotence in male (no flow in internal iliac vessels)

• Bilateral absent femoral and distal pulses

• Aortoiliac bruit.

d. How severe is the claudication?

Your examiner will almost certainly ask how you would manage your patient. This is influenced by your assessment of the severity of your patient's claudication. Use the following parameters:

• What is the claudication distance?

• Can your patient walk *through* the pain?

• How is it affecting your patient's lifestyle or work? (How far does he or she *need* to walk?)

• Has your patient tried conservative measures, eg stopping smoking, losing weight, an exercise programme?

• How rapidly is the problem progressing?

Treatment: if patient can actively enjoy life, leave well alone (90% managed conservatively); if not, consider arteriography and percutaneous dilation (the more proximal the disease the better the result).

Case 2: rest pain/critical ischaemia

The patient will usually be male, aged 60 +. A strong clue that he has rest pain is if his knee is bent or if his leg is hanging over the bed. Both these positions ease the pain. The following features differentiate rest pain from claudication:

- The pain is distal, mainly in the toes and forefoot
- Skin pallor
- Trophic changes (see page 209)
- Ischaemic ulceration at pressure points (see page 54)
- Gangrene: usually dry and wrinkled
- Positive Buerger's test (see page 211).

You may be asked why the pain occurs particularly at rest. There are three reasons:

1. Decreased arterial flow due to decreased assistance of gravity
2. Physiological decreased cardiac output at rest
3. Reactive dilatation of skin vessels to warmth (in bed).

Treatment: pain needs to be managed. Arteriogram is used to assess whether it is possible to dilate arterial stenosis, whether surgical reconstruction is possible and whether the patient is fit for surgery.

Case 3: diabetic foot

As in the above case, your patient may have ulcers at pressure points and gangrenous toes. Remember that the pathology is multifactorial:

- Arterial occlusive disease
- Microscopic angiopathy

- Peripheral neuropathy (sensory, motor, autonomic)

- Infection.

The following features distinguish the diabetic foot from the critically ischaemic foot:

- The patient is younger.

- The foot is red and warm.

- Gangrene is usually accompanied by infection: there may be deep collections of pus.

- The pulses may be present.

Treatment: treat infection. Neuropathic ulcers, with no ischaemia or acute infection – broad-spectrum antibiotics and follow the bone changes with MRI. May require conservative surgery to drain pus and remove dead tissue. May need more aggressive approach, as in Case 2.

Case 4: aortic aneurysm

This is a common short and long case in surgical finals. As always, look carefully. You may see a pulsating mass in the umbilical region.

An aortic aneurysm has an expansile pulsatility as opposed to a transmitted pulsatility. To distinguish between these, place the fingers of your two hands on either side of the mass and look to see if they are actually being pushed apart.

Measure the horizontal distance between your fingers: remember that, especially in thin females, the abdominal aorta is easily palpable.

Can your hand get above it? If so, it is infrarenal (most common).

Is the aneurysm tender? This suggests that it may be about to rupture (a very unlikely examination situation!).

Auscultate over the swelling: a loud bruit (in the absence of a similar bruit in the heart) supports the diagnosis.

Check the femoral, popliteal and foot pulses. These are usually present, as patients presenting with aneurysms rarely have peripheral vascular disease. However, emboli from the aneurysm may cause distal occlusion. There may be an associated popliteal aneurysm.

Treatment: when the aneurysm is >5.5 cm across (symptomatic or rapidly expanding), the risk of rupture continues to rise; if the patient is otherwise fit, the aneurysm should be replaced with a synthetic tube, using percutaneous (EVAR: endovascular aneurysm repair) or open surgical techniques.

Case 5: amputation

Peripheral vascular disease is by far the most common cause of amputation in elderly people. You might meet such a patient in the long case.

Take a detailed history of the immediate events leading up to the amputation but do not get bogged down in the probably lengthy history of previous operations such as bypasses and sympathectomies.

Your history should be geared largely towards the sociological implications of the amputation. Ask about mobility: can the patient climb stairs? Is he or she likely to be confined to a wheelchair? Assess the patient's ability to wash, dress and self-care in other ways. Ask also about occupational therapy, home help, aids and appliances.

Determine whether the amputation is below knee/through knee/above knee and look carefully at the wound site. Is it infected? Are there contractures of the hip and knee joints?

Treatment: vascular amputees need a wheelchair even where a prosthesis is proposed. Check whether the patient's home needs to be adapted: wheelchair accessibility is required for toilet and bathroom, reaching light switches, washing and cooking facilities, cupboards and getting onto their bed.

FAQS AND POPULAR VIVA QUESTIONS

1. Why does critical ischaemia lead to rest pain?

2. What is the cause of a bruit?

3. What factors would influence your management of a patient with claudication?

4. What are the causes of diabetic foot disease?

5. What causes of intermittent claudication would you consider in a young patient?

6. What are the causes of an acutely ischaemic limb?

7. What are the symptoms and signs of an acutely ischaemic limb?

8. What is the ankle–brachial pressure index (ABPI)? Why measure it?

9. What anatomical features on the arteriogram determine the severity of ischaemia in an atherosclerotic limb?

10. What are the risk factors for peripheral vascular disease?

ANSWERS

1. The blood supply is insufficient to keep the tissues alive; ischaemic metabolites and associated ulceration produce pain.

2. Turbulence when blood encounters a narrowing. High flow (associated with arteriovenous fistulae) can produce a bruit or a continuous murmur (machinery murmur). Murmurs can be transmitted from the heart, particularly to the carotid vessels.

3. (a) The effect on lifestyle: how far they can and need to walk, interference with work activities and social life; (b) response to preventive measures, eg stopping smoking, reaching an optimal weight and regular exercise; and (c) the rate of progress.

4. In diabetes, arterial disease occurs a decade earlier than in the rest of the population and is complicated by microvascular disease, neuropathy of motor or sensory and autonomic fibres, and increased susceptibility to infection.

5. Early onset of arteriosclerosis occurs in hyperlipidaemia, antiphospholipid syndrome, a bad family history, diabetes, someone who is a heavy smoker and Buerger's disease. Also consider compartment syndromes, popliteal entrapment and cystic degeneration, arterial injury and congenital anomalies, and exclude pain of neurological origin.

6. Trauma, embolism and thrombosis of aneurysms or pre-existing chronic disease.

7. The 6 Ps: pain, paraesthesia, paralysis, pallor, pulselessness, perishingly cold.

8. The ABPI is the ratio of the ankle to the arm blood pressure – usually >1 because the muscle bulk of the leg gives slightly higher readings. The value is reduced in lower limb arterial disease with a further fall on exercise.

9. Leg disease commonly starts in the superficial femoral artery at the adductor hiatus or its origin. Symptoms become prominent once disease is present at two levels, such as with additional popliteal or aortoiliac stenosis.

10. Family history, hyperlipidaemia, diabetes, smoking and hypertension.

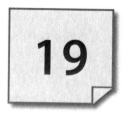

19   Venous disorders of the lower limb

THE HISTORY

Include the following questions.

Presenting complaint

- What is your main problem? (The patient may be bothered by the appearance, aches and pains or something else.)

- Are you on your feet all day? Do your legs ache more towards the end of the day?

- How long have you had the problem? Have you seen anyone about it previously? Was it treated then?

Predisposing causes

- Does anyone else in your family have varicose veins?

- Have you ever been pregnant? Did you have any problems with your legs then? Did one leg swell up?

- Have you had any major injuries or operations? Did you have any problems with your legs then? Did one leg swell up?

In your systemic enquiry, ask about abdominal and gynaecological symptoms, particularly,

- Have your noticed any swelling of your abdomen?

- Have your clothes become tighter lately?

THE EXAMINATION

Venous insufficiency is a common short case. Practise the tourniquet test. It may look easy on paper but the only way it doesn't end up an embarrassing fiasco in front of your examiners is for it to be a well-worn routine. Be absolutely clear about its significance. You may think that you understand it but, with exam nerves, explaining it is another matter. If you are being examined by a vascular unit, ask for a hand-held Doppler to test incompetence before performing the tourniquet test.

'Examine this patient's varicose veins'

ACTION	NOTE
Introduce yourself	
Say what you wish to do	
Ask the patient's permission to proceed	
Expose both legs with the patient standing up	
LOOK	
Compare shape of legs	*?beer-bottle leg*
Observe:	*?distribution of varicose veins* (long or short saphenous)
• anteriorly	
• posteriorly	
Observe skin changes in 'gaiter area' (lower third of leg, especially above medial malleolus)	*?venous stars* *?eczema* *?pigmentation* *?ulcers*

ACTION	NOTE
FEEL	
Run the back of your hand down both legs	*?warm over varicose veins*
Palpate along the medial side of the lower leg	
Ask if it is tender	*?tenderness* (occurs at sites of perforators)
Feel around the ankle	*?dermatoliposclerosis*
	?pitting oedema
Feel the saphenofemoral junction (4 cm below and lateral to pubic tubercle)	*?saphena varix*
Ask patient to cough	*?cough impulse* (indicates saphenofemoral incompetence)
Feel the saphenopopliteal junction (popliteal fossa)	
Ask patient to cough	*?cough impulse* (indicates saphenopopliteal incompetence)

ASSESS FURTHER

a. Tap test

Place the fingers of one hand at the lower limit of a long varicose vein	
Tap on the superial path of the vein with your other hand	*?percussion impulse* (indicates incompetence of *superficial* veins)

b. Tourniquet test

Ask patient to lie down flat	
Elevate one leg until the superficial veins are emptied	

ACTION	NOTE
Place a rubber tourniquet tightly around the upper thigh (if patient is unable to hold up leg, ask the examiner to hold it up)	
Ask patient to stand up	*?filling of superficial veins below tourniquet* (indicates incompetent perforators *below* tourniquet)
Watch *below* the tourniquet	
Keep repeating the procedure, moving the tourniquet progressively down the leg	
Position the tourniquet in between the sites of the perforator veins (see page 228)	
Repeat until the veins *below* the tourniquet stay collapsed	Defines the segment of leg containing incompetent perforators
c. Trendelenburg test for varicose veins	
Ask patient to lie flat	Perform this test only if the tourniquet test is positive at upper third of thigh
Elevate the leg until the superficial veins are emptied	
Place two fingers at the saphenofemoral junction	
Ask patient to stand up, keeping your fingers firmly in place	*?no filling of superficial veins below fingers ?filling on release of finger pressure* (indicates saphenofemoral incompetence)
Watch leg	

ACTION	NOTE
d. Perthes' test	
Place a tourniquet around the elevated leg so that the veins below tourniquet are empty	
Ask patient to stand up and down on tiptoe ten times	*?filling of superficial veins on exercise* (indicates deep venous occlusion)
Watch leg	
e. Listen	
Auscultate over sites of marked venous clusters	*?bruit* (indicates AV malformation – rare)
SAY	
'I would like to:	
• examine the abdomen	*?abdominal or pelvic mass* (cause may be inferior vena caval obstruction) (in females)
• do a rectal examination	
• do a pelvic examination	
• examine the external genitalia (in males)'	
If given a hand-held Doppler, kneel before the standing patient, place gel and probe over the short saphenous junction and compress the calf – normal whoosh upwards; incompetence also whoosh backwards	

COMPLETE THE EXAMINATION

Lie the patient down

Cover the legs

Turn to your examiner and present your findings

TYPICAL CASES

Although a patient with an acute deep vein thrombosis is unlikely to come up in an examination, you should know about the presentation and differential diagnosis of this common emergency.

Be absolutely clear as to what is meant by the terms 'varicose veins' and 'venous insufficiency'. Your patient may have one or both of these conditions.

Case 1: varicose veins

Your patient will usually have primary varicose veins, ie no known underlying cause. There may be a positive family history. However, always seek a secondary cause (see history and examination above).

You may be asked to define varicose veins: these are 'dilated, tortuous, thin-walled, superficial veins'.

A knowledge of the anatomy will help in your description of the distribution of the varicosities. Note that the muscular wall usually prevents dilation of the *main* leg veins: varicosities occur in the *tributaries*.

a. The long saphenous vein:

- Arises from the dorsal venous arch

- Runs anterior to the medial malleolus

- Runs behind the medial aspect of the knee

- Runs up the leg superficial to deep fascia

- Pierces cribriform fascia at the saphenous opening

- Empties into the femoral vein.

b. The short saphenous vein:

- Arises from the dorsal venous arch

- Runs behind the lateral malleolus

- Runs up the midline of the calf superficial to deep fascia

- Pierces deep fascia over the popliteal fossa

- Empties into the popliteal vein.

c. The perforator veins

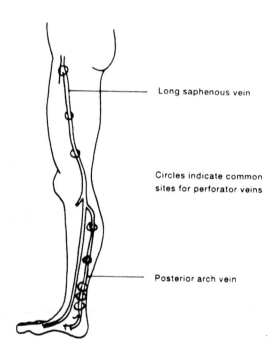

Long saphenous vein

Circles indicate common
sites for perforator veins

Posterior arch vein

Treatment:

1. Conservative measures with compression therapy with supportive hosiery and leg elevation.

2. Sclerotherapy of small varicosities (only after saphenous reflux has been excluded/treated) by injection of sclerosants.

3. Surgery is indicated if the patient has uncontrolled symptoms, venous ulceration or significant cosmetic concerns. This involves ligation of the saphenofemoral junction, great saphenous vein stripping, with avulsion of small varicosities below the knee.

4. Endovascular laser therapy (EVLT) and endovascular radiofrequency ablation of the great saphenous vein using ultrasound guidance. This has comparable results to saphenous vein stripping, but long-term recurrence rates need to be established.

Case 2: venous insufficiency

This describes the following dermatological course:

- Eczema (a low-grade cellulitis)

- Pigmentation (haemosiderin deposition)

- Venous ulcers (see page 53).

Your examiner will want to know if you have a clear understanding of the difference between *superficial* and *deep* venous insufficiency.

	Superficial venous insufficiency	Deep venous insufficiency
Aetiology	Primary varicose veins (unknown cause)	A late complication of deep vein thrombosis
Pathogenesis	Incompetent *perforator* veins: cause blood flow from *deep* to *superficial* system	Incompetent deep veins: lead to *raised pressure* in deep system. This causes blood flow from deep to *superficial* system (note that associated incompetent perforators can lead to *secondary* varicose veins)
Skin changes	Mild	Severe: 'beer-bottle leg' due to: • brawny oedema • dermatoliposclerosis (subcutaneous fat replaced by collagen)
Prognosis	Better response to surgery	Worse response to surgery

Treatment: conservative measures, with elevation of legs whenever convenient and supportive/compression hosiery.

Case 3: AV malformations

Although AV malformations are rare, they are lifelong problems, often with good physical signs, and they may therefore turn up as short cases.

Consider this diagnosis if you come across an easily compressible, superficial mass of vessels.

The malformation may be *congenital* or *acquired*. In a *congenital* AV malformation, your patient will tell you that the symptoms have been present from birth or childhood. There will often be gigantism of the affected limb. In *acquired* AV fistulae, there is a history of trauma. This may be surgically induced, as in the case of a fistula for haemodialysis.

Look for the following features:

- Signs of venous insufficiency

- Pulsatility

- Hum: always *listen* over large, unusually sited collections of varicosities.

Treatment: difficult as tend to recur. Injection of sclerosant into centre of malformation, usually via an arterial catheter; however, if this is not possible, transcutaneously into (or smaller amounts around) the vessels. Surgical excision of localised malformation involving non-essential tissue, more aggressive management if the lesion is affecting vision or hearing, or if cosmetically unacceptable.

FAQS AND POPULAR VIVA QUESTIONS

1. Describe the aetiology of varicose veins.

2. What do you understand by the term 'venous insufficiency'?

3. What are the indications for operating on a person with varicose veins?

4. How does an acute deep venous thrombosis present?

5. What are the causes of deep venous thrombosis?

6. What are the complications of a deep venous thrombosis?

ANSWERS

1. Varicose veins are superficial, thin-walled, elongated, tortuous, dilated veins. They may be primary congenital in origin, when there is often a family history. Both primary and secondary varicose veins are associated with valvular incompetence of the superficial system. Secondary varicose veins are associated with disease of the deep veins, eg previous deep vein thrombosis giving rise to superficial venous hypertension. Varicose veins may also be associated with arteriovenous malformations and fistulae.

2. Venous insufficiency describes a failure of the normal venous circulation: valves direct blood from the superficial to the deep vessels and from there, propelled by muscle pumps, back to the heart. It is associated with venous hypertension causing swelling and aching of the legs, particularly at the end of the day, and progressive skin changes – eczema, pigmentation, bleeding thrombosis, lipodermatosclerosis and ulceration.

3. Injection and/or surgery is indicated when the cosmetic appearance or the discomfort of the primary veins or their complications is unacceptable to the patient.

4. There are no symptoms in 50% of patients with deep venous thrombosis, or noted post-pulmonary embolism. The most common symptoms are a pale, swollen lower leg, calf tenderness, and pain on active and passive plantar- and dorsiflexion. If thrombosis extends enough to impair venous return, a blue swollen leg can lead to necrosis of superficial tissues; venous gangrene has a 50% amputation rate.

5. Thrombosis is produced by damage to the vessel wall, stasis or alteration in the constituents of the blood. These are all present after surgery and also when the patient is confined to bed. Hormonal changes also predispose to deep vein thrombosis, eg in association with the oral contraceptive pill, pregnancy, puerperium, hormonal replacement therapy. Thrombophlebitis is associated with serious illness, particularly malignancy.

6. Venous gangrene, pulmonary embolism and late sequelae of long-term venous insufficiency.

Neurology

20

Chronic neurological cases usually form part of medical finals, but the cranial nerves can be damaged by trauma and surgery, and sensory loss, and muscle wasting and weakness are easily missed if not routinely checked in every limb examination. This section considers surgically-related pathology.

Examination of the cranial nerves

The instruction may be to 'examine this patient's cranial nerves', or may be limited to one (perhaps VII or XII). If all, look around to see what equipment has been laid out for you, and talk the examiner through the procedure, because you may not be expected to examine them all and, with the simple statement of what you intend to do, you may be asked to proceed to the next nerve or you may also be asked to comment on the cause of any defect.

ACTION	NOTE
Introduce yourself	
Say what you wish to do	
Ask the patient's permission to proceed	
Sit the patient on the side of the bed or on a chair facing you	
Expose the head and neck to below the clavicles	
I Olfactory	
Test each nostril (ask patient to compress other side) with clove oil, peppermint, fetid odour (not pungent – stimulates V)	anosmia (loss of smell): *fractures across cribriform plate*

ACTION	NOTE
II Optic	
Test pupillary reflexes, visual fields and visual acuity	loss of pupillary and consensual response, and vision: *orbital trauma and monocular blindness*
ophthalmoscopy	homonymous hemianopia: *suprasellar tumour*
	bitemporal hemianopia: *disease of optic tract, radiation and cortex*
III Oculomotor	
Shine light into pupil, eye movements (combined III, IV, V)	loss of direct pupillary and contralateral consensual response, dilated pupil, diplopia: *trauma to orbit and middle cranial fossa, raised intracranial pressure*
IV Trochlear	
Test eye movements	loss of downward gaze (superior oblique): *trauma to orbit and middle cranial fossa*
VI Abducent	loss of lateral gaze (lateral rectus): *trauma to orbit and middle cranial fossa, raised intracranial pressure*
Test eye movements	remember LR6 SO4
V Trigeminal	loss of corneal reflex, loss of sensation over face, weakness of muscles of mastication: *trauma and surgery to facial region*
Test corneal reflex, sensation on face, teeth and gums; test bite to feel temporalis and masseter	
VII Facial	
Ask patient to smile, whistle, blow out cheeks and show teeth; check taste	total facial paralysis: *fractured base of skull, parotid disease and surgery*

ACTION	NOTE
	lower facial paralysis: *upper motor neurone lesion*, loss of taste on anterior tongue
VIII Acoustic	
Check hearing – whisper, Weber's test; Rinne's teat	loss of hearing, tuning fork heard only in good ear: *fractured skull base, acoustic tumours*
IX Glossopharyngeal	
Check gag reflex	loss of gag reflex: *skull base tumours*
X Vagus	
Ask patient to cough and observe soft palate when they say 'ah'	vocal fold paralysis, deviated uvula: *skull base tumours*
XI Accessory	
Ask patient to protrude jaw and shrug shoulders; repeat against resistance (and turning chin to the good side against your hand)	paralysis of sternomastoid and trapezius: *trauma and surgery to posterior triangle of neck*
XII Hypoglossal	
Ask patient to put out the tongue and push it against cheek; repeat against your pressure on the outside of the cheek	paralysis and protrusion towards damaged side: *laceration, surgery and tumours in the region of the carotid bifurcation*

Examination of the peripheral nervous system

Examination of the peripheral nervous system is not usually part of surgical finals, but it is repeatedly emphasised that, in every limb (and major joint) examination, you should check peripheral sensation (and pulses) and note muscle wasting. The following scheme is for sensory testing of the upper limb. Upper limb nerve injuries are considered with the hand (see page 194) and lower limb neurological testing with examination of the limb (see page 152). Upper limb sensory testing (with eyes closed) of dermatomes (individual nerves, see page 191).

ACTION	NOTE
Introduce yourself	
Say what you wish to do	
Ask the patient's permission to proceed	
Expose both upper limbs, including shoulders	
Sensory testing:	C4 shoulder; C5 lateral elbow; C6 thumb; C7 middle finger (variable); C8 little finger; T1 medial elbow
Touch (cotton wool) – first demonstrate with eyes open: 'Say yes every time you feel me touch you'	
Repeat above for **pain** (sterile needle or broken end of wooden stick – 'Is this sharp?') and **temperature** (side of finger vs cold side of tuning fork or test tubes of warm and cold water – 'Is it hot or cold?')	
Vibration – base of vibrating tuning fork on head of ulna: 'Say when it stops'	
Graphaesthesia – write numbers on forearm with a blunt instrument	
Stereognosis – recognising coin by touch	
Position sense – recognising direction of movement – hold sides of index finger and first demonstrate: 'This is up and this is down'	
Motor testing:	
Power – grip my fingers (offer just index and middle); bend your elbow (C5 and C6); straighten your arm (C7 and C8); small muscles of hand (T1)	

ACTION	NOTE
Tone – passive flexion and extension of relaxed elbow joint	
Coordination – finger to tip of nose – eyes open and then closed	
Reflexes – biceps C5 and C6; supinator, triceps C6 and C7	
Note wasting and abnormal movements	
Individual muscles – active and passive movements, and against resistance	

POPULAR VIVA QUESTIONS

1. What is the Glasgow coma scale (GCS)?

2. What do you mean by coning?

3. How do you differentiate between a runny nose and a CSF leak?

4. What is a pseudobulbar palsy?

5. What are the causes of a homonymous hemianopia?

6. What are the features of a facial palsy?

7. What are the features of a hypoglossal nerve injury?

8. What brachial plexus injuries would you expect from a motorcycle accident?

9. What is Tinel's sign?

10. What are the features of a femoral nerve palsy?

ANSWERS

1. The **Glasgow coma scale** is a system for assessing cerebral damage following a head injury – it scores eye, verbal and motor performance, E + V + M: minimum = 3, maximum = 15

Response	Details	Score
Best eye response (E)	Eyes open spontaneously	4
	Eyes opening to verbal command	3
	Eyes opening to pain	2
	No eye opening	1
Best verbal response (V)	Orientated	5
	Confused	4
	Inappropriate words	3
	Incomprehensible sounds	2
	No verbal response	1
Best motor response (M)	Obeys commands	6
	Localising pain	5
	Withdrawal from pain	4
	Flexion to pain	3
	Extension to pain	2
	No motor response	1

A GCS of 13 or higher correlates with a mild brain injury; 9–12 is a moderate injury; and 8 or less is a severe brain injury (the components should be presented with the score).

2. **Coning** is associated with raised intracranial pressure, the brain being compressed through the opening of the tentorium cerebelli or the foramen magnum. Early signs are pupillary changes (initial stimulation giving constriction, and then paralysis and dilatation) and loss of upward gaze due to compression of the oculomotor nerve(s) against the free edge of the tentorium. The condition is usually fatal. Note that it can be precipitated by a lumbar puncture in the presence of raised intracranial pressure – always exclude papilloedema before undertaking the procedure, or perform a CT scan.

3. Leaking cerebrospinal fluid is distinguished from other clear nasal drips by its sugar content and, when mixed with blood, by a separate diffusion ring on filter paper.

4. **A bulbar palsy** is produced by damage to the cranial nerve motor nuclei in the brainstem (mid- and hindbrain). However, these nuclei

receive a bilateral cortical innervation; thus unilateral cortical lesions (lesions of the upper motor neurone) produce no cranial nerve paresis (for an exception, see answer 6 below). Thus, to produce paralysis, cortical lesions have to be bilateral – when this occurs it is referred to as a **pseudobulbar palsy**.

5. A **homonymous hemianopia** is loss of vision to one side of the body (the ipsilateral nasal retina and contralateral lateral retina). To produce this defect, the lesion is posterior to the crossing in the optic chiasm, ie in the optic tract, radiation or cortex. Lesions anterior to the chiasm affect only one eye; lesions at the chiasm (eg pituitary tumours) compress the crossing fibres of both sides, producing a bitemporal hemianopia.

6. A lesion of the facial nerve nucleus in the pons or the nerve itself (ie a lower motor neurone lesion) produces complete facial paralysis. The usual surgical causes are parotid tumours, their surgical management and Bell's disease. Only part of the nucleus is bilaterally innervated (see answer 4 above) and in a stroke patient, the lower face is paralysed but the upper face is spared.

7. The **hypoglossal nerve** innervates the tongue and damage to the nerve produces wasting and weakness; on protrusion the tongue is deviated towards the affected side. The nerve may be damaged by infiltrating malignancies of the pharynx and surgery in the region of the carotid bifurcation. Unilateral cortical lesions do not affect tongue movements.

8. The classic motorcycle injury of the **brachial plexus** is avulsion of the upper (C5,6) roots (the helmet is in contact with the road and the shoulder is pulled downwards, stretching that side of the neck). There is loss of elbow flexion and supination. The limb hangs down the side, with palm facing backwards (waiter's tip position). This Erb's palsy may also be encountered after a difficult forceps delivery at birth.

9. A divided or damaged peripheral nerve regenerates and, if unimpeded, growth is about 1mm/day. If the regenerating end is percussed a tingling is produced and this **Tinel's sign**, which is used as a way of monitoring progress.

10. Damage to the **femoral nerve** paralyses hip flexion and knee extension, and produces numbness over the anterior and medial thigh and along the saphenous distribution to the medial leg and foot. The injury can be caused by surgery around the psoas muscle and sheath; a profound temporary paresis can follow a spontaneous retroperitoneal bleed in patients on anticoagulants.

21 The postoperative patient

Surgical wards have a high proportion of postoperative patients who are readily available for examinations. Patients who have recently undergone vascular, gastrointestinal or transplant surgery may come up as long cases.

In any part of the clinical examination expect questions on postoperative complications (eg pain, respiratory problems, wounds) and fluid balance. Familiarise yourself with bedside charts, which may be used as a basis for discussion and OSCEs.

THE HISTORY

Take a history of both the presenting complaint (ie circumstances that led up to this admission) and postoperative events. Screen for common postoperative complications by asking the following questions.

Pain

- Are you in any pain? (Ask specifically about leg pain, chest pain and increasing wound pain).

Respiratory symptoms

- Since the operation, have you:

  – been short of breath?

  – had a cough?

  – coughed up blood?

Gastrointestinal symptoms

- Have you passed a motion or flatus since the operation?
- Have you noticed any swelling of your abdomen?
- How is your appetite?
- Are you able to eat normally?
- Do you have any nausea or vomiting?

Urinary symptoms

- Did you have a catheter?
- Have you passed urine since the operation?
- Have you had any difficulty passing urine?
- Is there any pain when you pass urine?

Ask also about drugs, including analgesics, antibiotics and heparin prophylaxis.

Take a detailed social history: Does the patient live alone? Who will look after him or her after leaving hospital? On which floor does the patient live: are there many stairs to climb/do the lifts work?

THE EXAMINATION

When you examine a postoperative patient, first take a note of the tubes and measuring devices around the bed. Then go on to examine the patient. Finally, never omit to look at observation, fluid and drug charts that will probably be available.

Follow the scheme opposite.

'Examine this postoperative patient'

ACTION	NOTE
Introduce yourself	
Say what you wish to do	
Ask the patient's permission to proceed	
LOOK AROUND THE BED	
• Drips	*?number*
	?sites
	?fluid type
	?rate of delivery
• Lines	*?central venous line*
	?arterial line
• Drains	*?number*
	?site
	bag contents: *?amount*
	?colour
	?blood
	seal: *?sealed unit*
	?underwater seal
• Nasogastric tube	bag contents: *?amount*
	?colour
• Urinary catheter	*?open bag*
	?wash-out attachment
	?volume of urine
	?blood in urine

ACTION	NOTE
EXAMINE PATIENT	
a. Preliminary assessment	
Form a general impression of the patient	?ill
	?in pain
	?evidence of recent weight loss
	?hydration status
Check the mental state	?oriented in time/place/person
Look at the hands	?pale skin creases (clinically anaemic)
	?muscle wasting
	?loss of skin turgidity on back of hand (dehydration)
Take the pulse	
Take the blood pressure	
Look at the eyes	?sunken (dehydration)
Look at the conjunctivae	?pale (clinically anaemic)
Look at the sclerae	?jaundice
Pinch skin on abdomen	?lack of skin turgor (dehydration)
b. Examine the chest	signs of: ?infection
	?atelectasis
	?fluid overload
	?dehydration
c. Examine the abdomen (pages 100–104)	Ileus can lead to absent bowel sounds after abdominal or retroperitoneal surgery

ACTION	NOTE
d. Examine the wound	?site
	?type
	?stitches/clips
	?apposition of edges
	?redness
	?swelling
	?bruising
	?discharge
e. Examine the legs	?swelling
	?tenderness over calf
f. Examine the pressure areas	
• Sacrum	?bedsores
• Heels	
• Elbows	
LOOK AT THE CHARTS	
Temperature chart	?pyrexia
Nursing observations	?pulse
	?blood pressure
	?respiratory rate
Fluid balance	?input = output
Drug chart	?type of analgesia
	?drugs for medical problems
COMPLETE THE EXAMINATION	
Make sure that your patient is comfortable	
Turn to the examiner and present your findings	

FAQS AND POPULAR VIVA QUESTIONS

1. What is the normal daily requirement of water, sodium and potassium?

2. How would you determine the amount of fluid to prescribe in the first 24 hours after a laparotomy?

3. How would you assess dehydration/overhydration?

4. What is the difference between a crystalloid and a colloid?

5. What are the complications of blood transfusion?

6. Define oliguria.

7. How would you manage a patient with oliguria for more than 24 hours postoperatively?

8. How would you manage a patient with an increased pulse rate and drop in blood pressure postoperatively?

9. Tell me about prophylaxis against deep vein thrombosis.

10. What are the possible causes of a pyrexia between 2 and 10 days after surgery?

11. What are some of the alternatives for pain relief after surgery?

12. What are some of the predisposing factors for wound infection?

13. What are the respiratory complications after major surgery?

14. How would you manage a patient with (a) type 1 and (b) type 2 diabetes pre-, peri- and postoperatively?

ANSWERS

1. Normal requirements: 2.5–3 litres a day of water; 70 mmol of sodium (1–2 mmol/kg) and 60 mmol of potassium (1 mmol/kg).

2. Fluid loss (through aspiration via a nasogastric tube, diarrhoea, stoma output, vomiting, an intestinal fistula and sequestration of fluid into various body cavities) is added to the 2.5–3 litres of daily fluid requirement. However, precise measurement of urine output (a catheter being routinely used after major surgery) is documented on fluid balance charts, and also measured losses from other sites. These measurements are supplemented by clinical examination and other tests as described in the answer to question 3.

3. Signs of **dehydration** are a rising pulse, falling blood pressure, reduced capillary refill, decreased skin turgor, reduced urine output and falling jugular venous pressure (or central venous pressure when the line is in position). Serial measurement of blood urea and creatinine clearance may show progressive abnormality. Overhydration may be more difficult to diagnose. In a patient with good renal and cardiac function, urine output increases to maintain fluid balance but in elderly people the increased load can give rise to cardiac failure. Signs of **fluid overload** include peripheral oedema (usually over the sacrum in recumbent patients or dependent ankle oedema), pulmonary oedema as evidenced by basal crepitations, dyspnoea and a frothy sputum, pleural effusions, ascites and raised jugular venous pressure. Overload may be due to inappropriate amounts of 5% dextrose and may be associated with hyponatraemia.

4. The previous two answers have considered replacing appropriate volume and fluid loss. Attention is also given to the type of fluids prescribed. A typical prescription is 2 litres of 5% dextrose to every litre of dextrose/saline to satisfy daily requirements of sodium and carbohydrate. If the fluid loss is through haemorrhage, this may be replaced by blood transfusion. Attention may also be required to maintaining the circulating osmotic pressure of serum by prescribing a colloid solution, such as Haemaccel or human albumin. Colloid solutions are less likely than crystalloids to be rapidly excreted by the kidney. The logic of replacing circulating fluid loss with a similar constituent such as human albumin has not been consistently successful.

5. **Complications of blood transfusion** include acute immunological problems (after transfusing the wrong blood) with ABO and rhesus incompatibility, urticarial and anaphylactic reactions. Other immunological complications include transfusion-related acute lung injury and delayed reactions such as post-transfusion purpura, graft-versus-host disease and immunomodulatory effects. Non-immunological effects include hypothermia, hyperkalaemia, hypercalcaemia, congestive cardiac failure and iron overload. Infection can result from bacterial contamination of the transfusion apparatus or transfer from the donor (eg hepatitis B and C, HIV-I and -II, HTLV-I and -II (human T-lymphocytic virus), parvovirus, cytomegalovirus, malaria, babesiosis, brucellosis, trypanosomiasis and syphilis).

6. **Oliguria** is excretion of less than 400 ml of fluid over 24 hours.

7. **Management of oliguria** is dependent on the cause. Postrenal obstructive disease such as prostatic hyperplasia, bladder neck obstruction, stones and tumours must be relieved by catheterisation and appropriate management of the underlying cause. In renal failure, treatment is aimed at avoiding hyperkalaemia and retention of waste products. Glucose/insulin solutions may control hyperkalaemia but, with progressive disease, haemofiltration or haemodialysis may be required. In prerenal failure, fluid must be replaced. Rapid infusion may require a wide-bore central line, the volume being monitored by central venous or wedge pressures if a pulmonary artery line is in place. Aliquots of 150 ml of fluid can be delivered when the central venous pressure is <3 cmH$_2$O. It may be repeated until the level begins to rise. Other factors of overhydration, as described in (3), must also be undertaken to ensure that the reading is not a spurious one and that the quantity of fluid is appropriate.

8. A postoperative increase in pulse rate accompanied by a falling blood pressure indicates inadequate circulating blood volume, due to haemorrhage or fluid loss from other sources. Replacement is urgently required. Crystalloid is prescribed in the acute management and delivered rapidly in monitored aliquots. Blood is considered if haemorrhage is the cause and other causes addressed.

9. **Venous thrombosis** is a common postoperative complication. The thrombotic triad of stasis, damage to the vessel wall and alteration of blood constituents are all present (Virchow's triad). Some degree of calf thrombosis occurs in 50% of patients, probably starting at the

time of surgery, although clinically obvious DVT classically occurs at 7–10 days, as does pulmonary embolism. Prophylactic measures are therefore advisable, particularly in prolonged surgery and in high-risk groups such as those with previous DVTs, malignancy, obesity and age >40. Antithrombotic above-knee compression stockings are appropriate in all major surgery. Additional prophylactic measures include calf pneumatic compression devices and subcutaneous low molecular weight heparin.

10. **Fever** is defined as a temperature of >38°C. It is commonly related to **infection**, which may be present in the wound, respiratory and urinary tracts, uterus or skin. Abdominal surgery is particularly associated with peritonitis from leakage of gut flora. Bacteraemia may also give rise to cannula infections: particularly susceptible individuals are young and old people, people with alcohol problems, and patients with cardiac valvular disease, diabetes or immunosuppression. **Non-infective causes of pyrexia** include atelectasis, DVT, haematoma formation, transfusion reactions, myocardial infarction, some tumours (eg renal), connective tissue disorders and drug reactions. Malignant intra-operative hyperthermia is an inherited response to suxamethonium.

11. **Pain** is an inevitable result of surgery. It may be background, continuous or breakthrough. Milder forms of pain, in patients who can take oral preparations, can be managed with paracetamol and non-steroidal anti-inflammatory drugs, opioids including codeine, dihydrocodeine, oxycodone and tramadol. For more severe pain, morphine is usually administered; this may be intravenous or intramuscular, or as a continuous, possibly patient-controlled, subcutaneous injection. Local anaesthetic can be injected into wounds at operation and epidural pain control is valuable when appropriate. Entonox is useful for short, painful procedures.

12. **Wound infection** may be inevitable when operating through a contaminated field and is increased if there is haematoma formation. Organisms may come from the skin, be blood-borne or come from the underlying infective sources, particularly in association with peritonitis.

13. The most common **respiratory complication** is infection. Dry gases and reduced ciliary movement produce debris and, together with oropharyngeal secretions, this predisposes to tracheobronchitis, pneumonia and acute respiratory distress syndrome. Atelectasis is

also common because ventilation is not uniform throughout the pulmonary tree under anaesthesia, and the debris causing infection may also block bronchi and bronchioles. Reduced postoperative ventilation may be due to diaphragmatic splinting or sedation, and is increased in those who smoke and patients with previous respiratory problems; pain also inhibits respiratory executions. Pneuomothorax may be due to hyperinflation and misplaced central lines. Pulmonary embolism may follow a DVT.

14. People with **diabetes** undergoing major surgery should be brought into hospital at least the night before surgery. Type 1 patients should be converted to short-acting insulin. In type 2, oral medication should be changed to a short-acting sulphonylureas. On the day of the surgery, an insulin-glucose infusion should be started. The concentrations will depend on the patient's expected requirement but typically 15 U in a 500-ml pack of 5% dextrose can deliver 3 U in 100-ml aliquots delivered over an hour. Concentrations are varied with hourly blood sugar estimations and potassium supplements can be added to the infusion.

INDEX

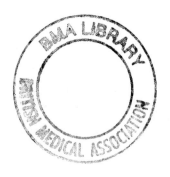